SUCCESS!

Phlebotomy

A Q&A Review

Sixth Edition

Kathleen Becan-McBride, EdD, MT(ASCP)
Director, Community and Educational Outreach
Coordinator, Texas–Mexico Border Health Services
Medical School Professor in the Department of Family and
Community Medicine
The University of Texas Health Science Center at Houston
Texas Medical Center, Houston, Texas
Assistant Director for Academic Partnerships, Greater Houston AHEC

Diana Garza, EdD, MT(ASCP)
Retired Professor, Health Sciences
Educational Consultant
Medical Writer/Editor
Houston, Texas

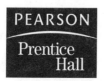

PEARSON
Prentice
Hall

Upper Saddle River, New Jersey 07458

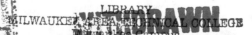

Library of Congress Cataloging-in-Publication Data

Becan-McBride, Kathleen
   SUCCESS! in Phlebotomy: A Q&A Review / Kathleen Becan-McBride, Diana Garza.— 6th ed.
      p. ; cm.
   Rev ed. of: Prentice Hall Health Q & A review for phlebotomy. 5th ed. c2001.
   Companion v. to: Phlebotomy handbook / Diana Garza, Kathleen Becan-McBride. 7th ed. c2005.
   Includes index.
   ISBN 0-13-118326-5
   1. Phlebotomy—Examinations, questions, etc.
   [DNLM: 1. Phlebotomy—Examination Questions.   QY 39 G245p 2005 Suppl. 2006]   I. Title: SUCCESS! in Phlebotomy: A Q&A Review.   II. Title: SUCCESS! in Phlebotomy: A Q&A Review.   III. Garza, Diana.   IV. Becan-McBride, Kathleen. SUCCESS! in Phlebotomy: A Q&A Review.   V. Garza, Diana. Phlebotomy handbook. VI. Title.
   RB45.15.G37 2005 Suppl.
   616.07′561—dc22

2005005096

Notice: The authors and the publisher of this volume have taken care that the information and technical recommendations contained herein are based on research and expert consultation and are accurate and compatible with the standards generally accepted at the time of publication. Nevertheless, as new information becomes available, changes in clinical and technical practices become necessary. The reader is advised to carefully consult manufacturers' instructions and information material for all supplies and equipment before use and to consult with a health care professional as necessary. This advice is especially important in using new supplies or equipment for clinical purposes. The authors and publisher disclaim all responsibility for any liability, loss, injury, or damage incurred as a consequence, directly or indirectly, of the use and application of any of the contents of this volume.

Publisher: Julie Levin Alexander
Publisher's Assistant: Regina Bruno
Executive Editor: Mark Cohen
Associate Editor: Melissa Kerian
Editorial Assistant: Jaquay Felix
Director of Manufacturing and Production: Bruce Johnson
Managing Editor for Production: Patrick Walsh
Production Editor: Karen Berry/Pine Tree Composition, Inc.
Manufacturing Manager: Ilene Sanford
Manufacturing Buyer: Pat Brown
Creative Director: Cheryl Asherman
Senior Design Coordinator: Maria Guglielmo-Walsh

Cover Designer: Anthony Gemmellaro
Director of Marketing/Marketing Manager: Karen Allman
Channel Marketing Manager: Rachele Strober
Marketing Coordinator: Michael Sirinides
Marketing Assistant: Patricia Linard
Media Editor: John Jordan
Media Production Manager: Amy Peltier
Media Project Manager: Stephen Hartner
Composition: Pine Tree Composition, Inc.
Printer/Binder: Courier Companies, Inc.
Cover Printer: Phoenix Color

Credits and acknowledgments borrowed from other sources and reproduced, with permission, in this textbook appear on appropriate page within text.

Pearson Education, LTD.
Pearson Education Singapore, Pte. Ltd.
Pearson Education, Canada, Ltd.
Pearson Education–Japan
Pearson Education Australia PTY, Limited

Pearson Education North Asia Ltd.
Pearson Educación de Mexico, S.A. de C.V.
Pearson Education Malaysia, Pte. Ltd.
Pearson Education, Upper Saddle River, New Jersey

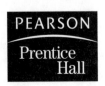

10 9 8 7 6 5 4 3 2 1
ISBN 0-13-118326-5

Contents

SECTION III: Phlebotomy Procedures 139

SECTION IV: Special Procedures and Point-of-Care Testing 191

Preface

The number of clinical laboratory techniques, automated instruments, and analyses continues to escalate, increasing the demand for proper collection of patient laboratory specimens. Since the majority of laboratory errors occurs in the preanalytical phase, it is essential that health care students and practitioners who are responsible for blood and specimen collections (i.e., phlebotomists, clinical laboratory technologists and technicians, nurses, respiratory therapists, and others) have an in-depth knowledge of their professional responsibilities. National board certification in phlebotomy is required by many health care institutions, clinics, and physicians' offices as a result of federal, safety, and quality assurance requirements. In addition, the rationale for phlebotomy state licensure is gaining momentum across the nation. Because of these laws and to ensure high-quality patient care, continuing education in phlebotomy safety and quality assurance has become paramount.

These important events in the responsibilities of blood collection have served to shape the sixth edition of *SUCCESS! in Phlebotomy.* It has been designed to act as a study companion for those who are (1) preparing for national or state board certification/licensure examinations and/or (2) pursuing self-assessment in blood collection.

SUCCESS! in Phlebotomy, **Sixth Edition,** includes 830 multiple-choice questions as a means to the overall review of blood collection, handling, and transportation. The chapters in this book are sequenced to match the order in *Phlebotomy Handbook: Blood Collection Essentials,* **Seventh Edition.** The question-and-answer content are divided into the following major sections:

- An Overview of the roles and functions of phlebotomists in the health care industry, legal issues, and the basics of anatomy and physiology with an emphasis on the cardiovascular system.
- Safety Procedures and Equipment provides information about safety and infection control in the workplace and the documentation and transportation procedures needed for safe handling of biohazardous specimens with comprehensive coverage on the latest blood collection equipment and supplies.
- Phlebotomy Procedures with the most updated questions and information on actual techniques used in blood collection and the clinical and technical complications that may occur in phlebotomy procedures.
- Special Procedures and Point-of-Care Testing, including information about pediatric phlebotomy procedures, arterial and IV collections, and special considerations for the elderly, homebound, and long-term care patients.

Each chapter includes chapter objectives as a guide. After the reader learns the essential topics in the *Phlebotomy Handbook: Blood Collection Essentials,* **Seventh Edition,** he or she can review them through the questions and answers presented in this book. Alternatively, this book may stand alone as a review book because it contains explanatory answers and the added feature of explanations for incorrect answers. These answers are all referenced to pages in the *Phlebotomy Handbook: Blood Collection Essentials,* **Seventh Edition,** so that the reader can obtain additional information on the question topic. This review book incorporates updated illustrations of blood collection equipment and techniques as bases for questions to help sharpen the phlebotomy skills. A corresponding Website located at *www.prenhall.com/review* features additional practice and resources.

Using the book will assist the reader in identifying areas of relative strength and weakness in the command of phlebotomy skills and responsibilities. After reviewing the multiple-choice questions and answers, the reader can practice taking the simulated examination provided on the accompanying CD. A diagnostic report identifies those topics that need further review and study.

SUCCESS! in Phlebotomy, **Sixth Edition,** *Phlebotomy Handbook: Blood Collection Essentials,* **Seventh Edition,** and the ***Instructor's Resource Guide with Test Bank and PowerPoint Lecture CD-ROM*** to accompany ***Phlebotomy Handbook*** are major *national* and *international* references for health care providers' educational programs, hospitals, physicians' offices, clinics, national examination boards, and legal issues in blood collection.

References

Garza, D., & Becan-McBride, K. (2005). *Phlebotomy Handbook: Blood Collection Essentials* (7th Edition). Upper Saddle River, NJ: Pearson/ Prentice Hall.

Kathleen Becan-McBride
Diana Garza

Introduction

SUCCESS!

ABOUT THE SUCCESS! SERIES

SUCCESS! is a complete exam preparation system that combines relevant exam-style questions with outline-style content review and interactive technology.

This format provides you with the best preparation for your exam!

- Build your experience & exam confidence!
- Practice with realistic exam-style questions.
- Enhance your review with state-of-the-art technology that offers more practice.

The **SUCCESS!** program is a proven method for increasing pass rates in many health professions from EMS to Nursing. We invite you to use our exam preparation system and HAVE SUCCESS!

Prentice Hall's complete **SUCCESS!** system includes review for the following areas:

Clinical Laboratory Science/Medical
   Technology
Dental Assisting

Dental Hygiene
Emergency Medical
   Services

Health Information Management
Home Health Aide
Massage Therapy
Medical Assisting
Nursing Assisting
Pharmacy Technician
Phlebotomy
Surgical Technology

Visit *www.prenhall.com/health* for more information on these or other Prentice Hall Health titles.

 ## ABOUT SUCCESS! IN PHLEBOTOMY

Part of the **SUCCESS!** Series, *SUCCESS! in Phlebotomy,* **Sixth Edition,** offers you a comprehensive approach to phlebotomy review. The question and answer review in the book, practice exam on the CD-ROM, and additional review and resources on the corresponding Website provide the practice needed for SUCCESS! on the ASCP, NPA, and NCA certification exams.

In the Book

Chapter Objectives

Each chapter opens with objectives that allow you to preview the topics covered. At a glance you will be able to identify the information and skills that you are responsible for knowing.

Realistic Exam-Style Questions

This review book contains 780 exam-style multiple-choice questions organized by topic area. Working through these questions will help you assess your strengths and weaknesses in each topic of study. These questions have been written at three different levels that consist of:

- *Recall*—the ability to recall previously memorized knowledge, skills, and facts
- *Applications*—the ability to apply recalled knowledge in verbal and written skills
- *Problem Solving*—the ability to apply recalled knowledge in solving a problem or case situation

Answers and Rationales

For each question in the book, answers are provided with rationales for both correct and incorrect responses allowing you to fully comprehend the answer.

References

Enhance your review by referencing ***Phlebotomy Handbook: Blood Collection Essentials,*** **Seventh Edition,** by Diana Garza and Kathleen Becan-McBride as you practice with ***SUCCESS! in Phlebotomy,*** **Sixth Edition.** Answers to all questions contained in ***SUCCESS! in Phlebotomy,*** **Sixth Edition,** also include references to the best-selling title ***Phlebotomy Handbook: Blood Collection Essentials,*** **Seventh Edition,** allowing you to easily find more information and in-depth information on a specific topic area.

On the CD-ROM

Included with the book is a FREE CD-ROM that features a 100-question practice exam and audio glossary. This CD-ROM will assist you in determining your strengths, weaknesses and further areas for study. Answers are provided for all test questions.

On the Website

Visit *www.prenhall.com/review* for additional practice questions, an audio glossary, and links to related resources. Designed to enhance your review, you will want to bookmark this site as you continue on your path to SUCCESS!

 ## CERTIFICATION

Each of at least six organizations currently has certification tests in phlebotomy. If you intend to apply for one or more of the certification examinations, determine which particular phlebotomy certification examinations are better known and/or accepted in your local community and state. Sometimes health care organizations have preferences for specific certifications and will adjust salaries accordingly. Likewise, local community colleges and universities can also provide recommendations about which certification examination to take.

Also, some states are pursuing licensing of phlebotomists, which is required if you intend to work in that state. As a fairly recent example, California requires state licensure for phlebotomists and requires certain training and experience requirements similar to the national board requirements.

The organizations listed below have an interest in promoting and improving the practice of phlebotomy. They differ slightly in their membership requirements, fees, member benefits, continuing education courses, and/or to the degree that they offer certification specifically for phlebotomists.

The American Society for Clinical Pathology (ASCP)

Board of Registry
P.O. Box 12277
Chicago, IL 60612-0277
312.738.1336 or 800.621.4142
www.ascp.org

The National Phlebotomy Association (NPA)

1901 Brightseat Road
Landover, MD 20785
301.386.4200
301.386.4203 (fax)
www.scpt.com/NationalPhlebotomyAssociation
.html

The American Society for Clinical Laboratory Science (ASCLS) and The National Credentialing Agency for Laboratory Personnel, Inc. (NCA)

NCA
P.O. Box 15945-289
Lenexa, KS 66285
913.438.5110
www.nca-info.org

ASCLS
7910 Woodmont
Avenue, Suite 530
Bethesda, MD 20814
301.657.2768
www.ascls.org

American Medical Technologists (AMT)

710 Higgins Road
Park Ridge, IL 60068-5765
847.823.5169 or 800.275.1268
847.823.0458 (fax)
www.amt1.com

American Society of Phlebotomy Technicians (ASPT)

P.O. Box 1831
Hickory, NC 28603
828.294.0078
828.327.2969 (fax)
www.aspt.org

National Healthcareer Association (NHA)

National Headquarters
134 Evergreen Place, 9th Floor
East Orange, NJ 07018
800.499.9092
973.678.7305 (fax)
www.nha2000.com

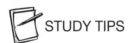 STUDY TIPS

Review Materials

Choose review materials that contain the information you need to study. Save time by making sure that you aren't studying anything you don't need to. Before the exam, the best study preparation would be to use this Question & Answer Review to identify your strengths and weaknesses. The references at the end of each rationale will direct you to additional resources for more in-depth study.

Set a Study Schedule

Use your time-management skills to set a schedule that will help you feel as prepared as you can be. Consider all the relevant factors—the materials you need to study, how many months, weeks, or days until the test date, and how much time you can study each day. If you establish your schedule ahead of time and write it in your date book, you will be much more likely to follow it.

Take Practice Tests

Practice as much as possible, using the questions in this book, on the accompanying CD, and the Web. These questions were designed to follow the format of questions that appear on the exam you will take, so the more you practice with these questions, the better prepared you will be on test day.

The practice tests on the CD will give you a chance to experience the exam before you actually have to take it and will also let you know how you're doing and where you need to do better. For best results, we recommend you take a practice test 2 to 3 weeks before you are scheduled to take the actual exam. Spend the next weeks targeting those areas in which you performed poorly by reviewing questions in those areas.

Practice under test-like conditions—in a quiet room, with no books or notes to help you, and with a clock telling you when to quit. Try to come as close as you can to duplicating the actual test situation.

TAKING THE EXAMINATION

Prepare Physically

When taking the exam, you need to work efficiently under time pressure. If your body is tired or under stress, you might not think as clearly or perform as well as you usually do. If you can, avoid staying up all night. Get some sleep so that you can wake up rested and alert.

Eating right is also important. The best advice is to eat a light, well-balanced meal before a test. When time is short, grab a quick-energy snack such as a banana, orange juice, or a granola bar.

The Examination Site

The examination site is usually selected at the time of registration and should be located prior to the required examination time. One suggestion is to find the site and parking facilities the day before the test. Parking fee information should be obtained so that sufficient money can be taken along on the examination day.

Allow plenty of time for travel to the site in case of unexpected mishaps such as traffic snarls. During travel, think positive thoughts (e.g., "My preparation for the exam was thorough, so I'll be able to answer the questions easily"). Maintain a confident attitude to prevent unnecessary stress.

Materials

Be sure to take all required identification materials (usually a photo ID), registration forms, and any other items required by the testing organization or center. Read information and instructions supplied by the testing organizations thoroughly to be sure you have all necessary materials (e.g., a non-programmable calculator) before the day of the exam. Do not carry textbooks or notes into the testing area. Scratch paper is often provided if needed. Remember, you will *not* be allowed to take the test if you forget any of the required forms or identification. And don't be surprised if you are fingerprinted and/or photographed when you enter the examination room. It is standard procedure at some testing centers to assure identity each time you enter and return to the room.

Read Test Directions

Read the examination directions thoroughly! Because some board examinations have different test sections with different question formats, it is important to be aware of changes in directions. Read each set of directions completely before starting a new section of questions.

Computerized Exams

To ensure that you are comfortable with the computer test format, be sure to practice on the computer using the CD-ROM that is included in the back of the book.

Since certification exam requirements vary, it is important to determine before taking a computerized exam whether you can change your answer after you strike a key for a particular answer. Checking your answers is a very important part of taking a major certification exam. Thus, do not enter an answer on a computerized exam unless you (1) have the option to change it as you are checking your answers or (2) are absolutely certain that your answer is correct when you first enter it.

During the exam, check the computer screen after an answer is entered to verify that the answer appears as it was entered. If you feel fatigued, close your eyes, take a few deep breaths, and stretch your arms and shoulders; then resume the examination. If you need assistance, check to see if there is a "HELP" function or contact the testing proctor.

Pencil and Paper Exams

Machine-scored tests require that you use a special pencil to fill in a small box on a computerized answer sheet. Use the right pencil (usually a No. 2), and mark your answers in the correct space. Neatness counts on these tests, because the computer can misread stray pencil marks or partially erased answers. Periodically, check the answer number against the question number to make sure they match. One question skipped can cause every answer following it to be marked incorrectly.

Selecting the Right Answer

Keep in mind that only one answer is correct. First read the stem of the question with *each* possible choice provided and eliminate choices that are obviously incorrect. Be cautious about choosing the first answer that *might* be correct; all possibilities should be considered before the final choice is made; the best answer should be selected. If a question is complicated, try to break it down into small sections that are easy to understand. Pay special attention to qualifiers such as *only, except,* etc. For example, negative words in a question can confuse your understanding of what the question asks ("Which of the following is *not* . . .").

Intelligent Guessing

If you don't know the answer, eliminate those answers that you know or suspect are wrong. Your goal is to narrow down your choices. Here are some questions to ask yourself:

- Is the choice accurate in its own terms? If there's an error in the choice, for example, a term that is incorrectly defined—the answer is wrong.
- Is the choice relevant? An answer may be accurate, but it may not relate to the essence of the question.
- Are there any distractors, such as *always, never, all, none,* or *every?* Qualifiers make it easy to find an exception that makes a choice incorrect.

Mark answers you are not sure of, and go back to them at the end of the test.

Ask yourself whether you would make the same guesses again. Chances are that you will leave your answers alone, but you may notice something that will make you change your mind—a qualifier that affects meaning or a remembered fact that will enable you to answer the question without guessing.

Watch the Clock

Keep track of how much time is left and how you are progressing. Wear a watch or bring a small clock with you to the test room. A wall clock may be broken, or there may be no clock at all.

Some students are so concerned about time that they rush through the exam and have time left over. In such situations, it's easy to leave early. The best approach, however, is to take your time. Stay until the end so that you can check your answers or, if the test is computerized, make sure you know how to "End" the test. Some exams provide a preliminary "Pass or Fail" result at the test site.

KEYS TO SUCCESS!

- Study, review, and practice
- Keep a positive, confident attitude
- Follow all directions on the examination
- Do your best

Good luck!

You are encouraged to visit http://www .prenhall.com/success for an additional practice exam and additional tips on studying, test-taking, and other keys to success. At this stage of your education and career you will find these tips helpful.

Some of the study and test-taking tips were adapted from Keys to Effective Learning, Second Edition, *by Carol Carter, Joyce Bishop, and Sarah Lyman Kravits.*

1

Phlebotomy Practice and Quality Essentials

chapter objectives

Upon completion of Chapter 1, the learner is responsible for the following:

➤ Define phlebotomy and identify health professionals who perform phlebotomy procedures.

➤ Identify the importance of phlebotomy procedures to the overall care of the patient.

➤ List professional competencies for phlebotomists and key elements of an employer's performance assessment.

➤ List skills for active listening and effective verbal communication.

➤ List examples of positive and negative body language.

➤ Describe health care settings where phlebotomy services are routinely performed.

➤ Give examples of how a phlebotomist can participate in quality improvement activities.

DIRECTIONS
Each of the questions or incomplete statements below is followed by four suggested answers or completions. Select one answer that is best in each case.

1. Most health care organizations fit into which of the following major categories of health care?
   A. specialty hospitals or clinics
   B. hospital or ambulatory care
   C. hospital or school based
   D. surgical centers or ambulatory centers

2. Job duties of phlebotomists can include which of the following:
   A. technical duties
   B. clinical duties only
   C. clinical, technical, and clerical duties
   D. technical and interpretive duties

3. Certification can provide advantages to phlebotomists in which of the following ways?
   A. automatic bonuses
   B. job opportunities, advancement, and portability
   C. improves accrued vacation time
   D. assures continuing education

4. The American Society for Clinical Pathology (ASCP), the National Phlebotomy Association (NPA), and the National Credentialing Agency for Laboratory Personnel (NCA) are examples of what type of organization?
   A. licensing
   B. quality control
   C. certification
   D. accreditation

5. The health care department that uses radioactive isotopes or tracers in the diagnosis and treatment of patients and in the study of the disease process is the:
   A. clinical laboratory department
   B. occupational therapy department
   C. diagnostic imaging/radiology department
   D. nuclear medicine department

6. Which of the following medical departments is associated with diagnostic and treatment procedures for bone and joint disorders and diseases?
   A. ophthalmology
   B. otolaryngology
   C. dermatology
   D. orthopedics

7. Which of the following departments deals with the general diagnosis and treatment of patients for problems of one or more internal organs?
   A. proctology
   B. anesthesiology
   C. internal medicine
   D. oncology

8. Which of the following sections is not part of the clinical laboratory?
   A. radiology
   B. chemistry
   C. microbiology
   D. hematology

9. Which of the following departments dispenses medications?
   A. clinical laboratory
   B. pulmonary

C. pharmacy

D. radiology

10. What type of diploma is required to enter most phlebotomy training programs?

A. high school or equivalent

B. associate degree

C. bachelor's degree

D. master's degree

11. Which of the following departments deals with health care for children?

A. pharmacy

B. clinical laboratory

C. radiology

D. pediatrics

12. A primary consultant on the timing for collecting blood for drug levels is found in which of the following departments?

A. pharmacy

B. nutrition and dietetics

C. occupational therapy

D. clinical hematology

13. Which of the following is an important method that all employers should use to provide an employee with feedback about their job and methods for improvement?

A. reprimands

B. a list of benefits

C. merit raises

D. performance evaluations

14. The following attributes of good judgment, respecting patients' rights, and not harming anyone intentialy are examples of which of the following?

A. ethical standards

B. confidentiality statements

C. competency statements

D. rules of practice

15. A medical doctor who usually has extensive education in the study and diagnosis of diseases through the use of laboratory test results is sometimes referred to as a:

A. medical laboratory technician

B. medical technologist

C. clinical laboratory scientist

D. pathologist

16. Which of the following departments deals with disorders affecting the organs and tissues that produce hormones?

A. neurology

B. otolaryngology

C. endocrinology

D. nephrology

17. Which of the following character traits is vitally important to phlebotomists?

A. personal integrity and veracity

B. quickness and speed writing

C. making rapid decisions

D. having strong mathematical skills

18. Which of the following departments is involved in the diagnosis and treatment of malignant tumors?

A. oncology

B. rheumatology

C. geriatrics

D. proctology

19. Phlebotomists must always work with which of the following?

A. personnel from the federal government

B. only the laboratory personnel

C. other members of the health care team

D. assigned physicians in the hospital

20. The department of gastroenterology refers to:
    A. nervous system
    B. ears, nose, and throat
    C. esophagus, stomach, and intestines
    D. organs and tissues that produce hormones

21. Mrs. J. Hamm, a patient who had blood tests requested from the nephrology department, probably has a disorder related to the:
    A. nervous system
    B. lungs
    C. kidneys
    D. immune system

22. Why is it important for phlebotomists to enjoy communicating with patients?
    A. improves public opinion
    B. is good for business
    C. helps Medicaid eligibility
    D. improves the likelihood of a successful patient interaction

23. Most hospital laboratory departments have which of the following?
    A. radiotherapy department
    B. emergency rooms
    C. anatomical or surgical pathology and clinical pathology
    D. pharmacy testing

24. Ambulatory care refers to health care services provided to:
    A. inpatients
    B. outpatients
    C. patients in acute care hospitals
    D. patients in long-term care hospitals

25. Which of the following is *not* an important purpose of laboratory analyses for a health assessment of an individual?
    A. monitoring of the patient's health status
    B. developing a community needs assessment
    C. diagnostic testing on the patient
    D. therapeutic assessment to develop the appropriate treatment

26. On the basis of recommended professional competencies for a certified phlebotomist, which of the following is a phlebotomist's professional competency?
    A. performs microscopic analysis of blood smears
    B. participates in the development of new laboratory testing instrumentation
    C. performs tests and records immunologic laboratory procedural results
    D. selects appropriate quality control procedures

27. Phlebotomists are primarily responsible for what phase of laboratory testing?
    A. preassessment
    B. preanalytical
    C. analytical
    D. post-analytical

28. All clinical laboratories are regulated by which of the following?
    A. Clinical Laboratory Improvement Amendments of 1988 (CLIA)
    B. American Association of Blood Banks (AABB)
    C. Medicaid
    D. Medicare

29. When a phlebotomist builds a good "rapport" with a patient, what is he or she doing?

   A. moving the patient to a different position for comfort

   B. being courteous and showing interest to improve patient satisfaction

   C. providing feedback about the illness

   D. filing lab reports in the patient's medical record

30. If a phlebotomist walks into a patient's room that has a television on very loudly, what should be the first course of action prior to beginning the procedure?

   A. Turn off the television immediately.

   B. Ask the patient if it is okay to reduce the volume or turn it off.

   C. Ignore it and proceed with the procedure because it distracts the patient from the pain of the venipuncture.

   D. Ask a family member to turn it off and step out of the room.

31. What should a phlebotomist do if a patient cannot speak English and the patient's 11-year-old child offers to translate for his parent during the initial patient encounter?

   A. Never allow the child to translate for his parent.

   B. Allow the child to translate during the critical parts of the procedure.

   C. Try to get a translator or written instructions in the patient's native language.

   D. Leave the room immediately without speaking to the patient so that the child will not misinterpret anything you say.

32. The clinical laboratory supervisor requested that Ms. Douglas, a phlebotomist, go quickly to the otolaryngology department to pick up a laboratory specimen belonging to Ms. Gonzales. The phlebotomist had to go to the department that provides treatment of the:

   A. eye

   B. ear, nose, and throat

   C. bones and joints

   D. skin

33. While setting up for a routine venipuncture, the patient asked the phlebotomist, "Will this hurt?" What is the most appropriate response?

   A. It doesn't hurt and only takes a few seconds anyway.

   B. It only hurts for one second.

   C. It will hurt a little, but it should be over quickly.

   D. It can be terribly uncomfortable for some patients, but for others it is a piece of cake.

34. Which of the following is the appropriate protocol for health care workers who are involved in specimen collection?

   A. Once the laboratory tests have been performed on a patient, the blood collector can discuss these with the patient and family.

   B. If the blood collector is a phlebotomy student, it is best not to inform the patient that he or she is a student, since it may make the patient nervous.

   C. If the family asked for information on their child's laboratory results, the blood collector should seek those results out to help the family.

   D. The blood collector should state that the patient's physician ordered blood to be collected for testing and that it would be best to discuss the laboratory tests with the physician.

35. If the phlebotomist collects blood in the neonatology department, what type of patient is he or she performing blood collections on?
    A. hours to a few days old
    B. 3 to 5 years old
    C. 1 to 3 years old
    D. pregnant patients

36. Which of the following is a term used for a health care worker with a 2-year degree who has specimen collection duties and may perform designated tests and procedures?
    A. occupational therapist (OT)
    B. medical laboratory technician (MLT)
    C. clinical laboratory scientist (CLS)
    D. physical therapist (PT)

37. For CLIA regulatory categories, which of the following are designated in the waivered tests category?
    A. bone marrow evaluation
    B. urine cultures
    C. urinalysis
    D. cytogenetics

38. A busy phlebotomist was in a hurry one morning when she quickly awakened her next patient and suddenly approached the patient for a routine venipuncture. The patient became visibly nervous, anxious, and refused to have her blood collected. Which of the following factors could explain the patient's reaction?
    A. The phlebotomist intruded into the patient's zone of comfort too quickly.
    B. The patient was overmedicated.
    C. This is normal procedure for approaching a patient and the patient's reaction was unjustified.

D. The phlebotomist was too cheerful and happy.

39. Cultural sensitivity for phlebotomists involves learning about all but which one of the following factors?
    A. values
    B. beliefs
    C. traditions and practices
    D. skin sensitivity to pain

40. In a health care setting, the "internal" customers include all but which one:
    A. physicians and medical students
    B. patients
    C. nurses and other allied health workers
    D. special interest groups

41. Which of the following behaviors should the phlebotomist avoid in his or her patient care and blood collection activities?
    A. making a deep sigh when collecting the blood
    B. smiling when he or she is around the patient
    C. making eye contact with the patient
    D. maintaining relaxed hands, arms, and shoulders

42. Which of the following departments in health care facilities has the specific responsibilities with diagnosis and treatment of the elderly population?
    A. geriatrics
    B. internal medicine
    C. psychiatry/neurology
    D. proctology

43. Which of the following patients' specimens would most likely be taken to anatomic pathology?

A. synovial fluid

B. biopsy tissue

C. cerebrospinal fluid

D. sputum

44. According to the Clinical Laboratory Improvement Amendments of 1988 (CLIA 88), the cytogenetics analysis and electrophoresis tests are considered to be:

A. waivered

B. extremely high-complexity

C. high-complexity

D. moderate-complexity

45. The PDCA cycle represents which of the following?

A. quality model for performing venipunctures

B. strategy for quality improvement to plan, do, check, and act

C. modified laboratory model

D. 10-step process for laboratory testing

46. Cause-and-effect diagrams can be used in quality improvement methodologies and are designed to assist in:

A. stimulating creative ideas

B. breaking out components into a flowchart

C. making bar charts that show the frequency of problems

D. identifying interactions between people, methods, equipment, and supplies

47. Pareto charts can be used in quality improvement methodologies and are designed to assist in:

A. making bar charts that show the frequency of problems

B. stimulating creative ideas

C. identifying interactions between people, methods, equipment, and supplies

D. breaking out components into a flowchart

48. Flowcharts can be used in quality improvement methodologies and are designed to assist in:

A. breaking out components into a diagram to understand a process

B. making bar charts that show the frequency of problems

C. stimulating creative ideas

D. identifying interactions between people, methods, equipment, and supplies

49. Quality improvement efforts for specimen collection frequently involve all but which one:

A. phlebotomist's technique

B. recollection rates

C. frequency of hematomas

D. negative drug reactions

50. Outcomes assessments for quality improvement include:

A. nosocomial infection rates

B. the presence of a pathologist 24 hours per day

C. the number of fire extinguishers available

D. all of the above

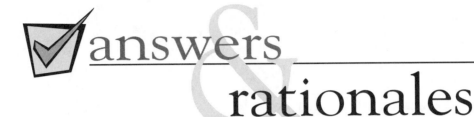

answers & rationales

1.

A. Specialty hospitals are usually devoted to only one type of disease or category of disorder while the term "clinic" is rather broad and refers to ambulatory care sites.

B. Most health care organizations in the United States fit into two major categories: hospital (inpatient) or ambulatory (outpatient) care. (p. 3)

C. Hospitals is one category, but school-based care is only pediatric care delivered on-site at school.

D. Surgical centers are usually restricted to day surgeries; ambulatory care is one of the major categories of health care.

2.

A. Technical duties involve selecting, preparing, and processing procedures related to phlebotomy. Phlebotomists do this and more.

B. Clinical duties involve identifying and assessing the patient, performing the venipuncture, and assessing the patient after the procedure. Phlebotomists do this and more.

C. Phlebotomists are often expected to perform clinical, technical, and clerical duties. (p. 6)

D. Interpretive duties are not included in a phlebotomist's job duties. Interpretation of laboratory results is the responsibility of the physician.

3.

A. While a few employers offer bonuses for passing a certification examination, it is not common practice; however, many employers require certification as a condition for employment.

B. Certification provides phlebotomists with career advantages through increased job opportunities, advancement opportunities, and portability (the ability to carry the certification from state to state). (p. 6)

C. Improving vacation time does not result from certification. This is a benefit that varies by employer.

D. Certification examinations do not assure continuing education; however, most certification agencies offer continuing education opportunities after passing a certification examination. Some states require continuing education for phlebotomists.

4.

A. Licensing is required by individual states; to date, most states do not require licensing for phlebotomists.

B. Quality control is a term used to describe the quality monitoring of supplies, reagents, and equipment.

C. ASCP, NPA, and NCA are examples of national certifying agencies that provide certification examinations for phlebotomists. (p. 7)

D. Accrediting agencies provide oversight and monitoring of health care organizations, not individuals.

5.

A. The clinical laboratory department uses instrumentation to analyze blood, body fluids, and tissues for pathological conditions.

B. The occupational therapy department assists the patient in becoming functionally independent within the limitations of the patient's disability or condition.

C. The diagnostic imaging/radiology department uses ionizing radiation for treating disease and fluoroscopic and radiographic x-ray instrumentation and imaging for diagnosis and treating disease.

D. The nuclear medicine department uses radioactive isotopes or tracers in the diagnosis and treatment of patients and in the study of the disease process. (p. 4)

6.

A. Ophthalmology is the department that has medical diagnosis and treatment for eye disorders.

B. Otolaryngology is the department that has medical diagnosis and treatment for ear, nose, and throat disorders.

C. Dermatology is the department that has medical treatments for skin disorders.

D. The orthopedics department performs diagnostic and treatment procedures for bone and joint disorders and diseases. (p. 5)

7.

A. Otolaryngology is the department that has medical diagnosis and treatment for ear, nose, and throat disorders.

B. Ophthalmology is the department that has medical diagnosis and treatment for eye disorders.

C. Internal medicine is the department involved in the general diagnosis and treatment of patients for problems of one or more internal organs. (p. 4)

D. Oncology is the department involved in the diagnosis and treatment of malignant tumors.

8.

A. The radiology department is not a part of the clinical laboratory. (pp. 5, 15)

B. Clinical chemistry is the section that performs analyses on blood to determine the level of chemical constituents such as glucose, cholesterol, and drugs, etc.

C. The clinical microbiology department performs analyses to detect microorganisms that are infecting the patient and include such tests as occult blood, blood cultures, and strep screening.

D. The hematology section performs analyses on blood to detect abnormal types and numbers of blood cells.

9.

A. The clinical laboratory performs analysis on blood and body fluids.

B. The pulmonary department provides diagnosis and treatment for disorders related to the respiratory tract.

C. The pharmacy dispenses medications ordered by physicians. Pharmacists collaborate with phlebotomists when monitoring drug levels. (p. 5)

D. The radiology department performs x-rays and ultrasonography as well as other imaging procedures.

10.

A. A high school diploma or its equivalent is most often required to enter a phlebotomy training program. (p. 3)

B. An associate degree is not required to enter most phlebotomy training programs.

C. A bachelor's degree is not required to enter phlebotomy training programs.

D. A master's degree is not required to enter phlebotomy training programs.

11.

A. Pharmacy departments dispense medications.

B. Clinical laboratories deal with analysis of blood and body fluids.

C. The radiology department performs x-rays and ultrasonography as well as other imaging procedures.

D. Pediatric departments deal with diagnosis and therapy for children. (p. 5)

12.

A. The pharmacy department dispenses medications ordered by the physician and collabo-

rates with the health care team on drug therapies. Typically, the clinical chemistry section works closely with the pharmacy dept on establishing correct timing for drug levels. (p. 5)**

B. The nutrition and dietetics department performs nutritional assessments, patient education, and designs special diets for patients who have eating-related disorders.

C. The occupational therapy department assists the patient in becoming functionally independent within the limitations of the patient's condition.

D. The clinical hematology department uses sophisticated instrumentation to analyze blood for pathological conditions.

13.

A. Reprimands are usually related to doing something wrong.

B. A list of benefits is usually provided when an employee is hired. It includes information about health insurance, etc.

C. Merit raises are sometimes given to employees for outstanding job performance.

D. Performance evaluations are important to both employees and employers because they provide feedback, identify problems that the employee may be having, promote consistency in the evaluation process, encourage employees to stay current, provide employees with improvement targets, and document that personnel are competent. (p. 9)

14.

A. These are examples of ethical standards of performance that are common to most professional organizations in the health care industry. (p. 9)

B. Confidentiality relates to not disclosing health care information that is private.

C. Competency statements relate to entry-level tasks and skills required by a job.

D. Rules of practice is not a phrase that is used in health care.

15.

A. A medical laboratory technician (MLT) has an associate's degree in the study of clinical laboratory testing and procedures.

B. A medical technologist (MT) usually has a bachelor's degree in a biological science with at least 1 year of study in a clinical laboratory science program.

C. A clinical laboratory scientist (CLS) is a medical technologist who has a bachelor's degree in a biological science with at least 1 year of study in a clinical laboratory science program.

D. A pathologist is a physician who has extensive training in pathology, which is the study and diagnosis of diseases through the use of laboratory test results. (p. 5)

16.

A. The neurology department deals with nervous system disorders.

B. The otolaryngology department deals with disorders of the ear, nose, and throat.

C. The endocrinology department deals with disorders affecting organs and tissues that produce hormones. (p. 4)

D. The nephrology department deals with renal (kidney) system disorders.

17.

A. Personal integrity and veracity involve telling the truth and doing things right when no one is looking. These traits are vitally important for a phlebotomist. (p. 9)

B. While quickness and speed writing can be helpful, they are not important traits when dealing with patients. It is more important to take time to perform duties carefully and thoroughly.

C. Making rapid decisions is helpful, but again, it is more important to take time to perform duties carefully, thoughtfully, and thoroughly.

D. Having strong math skills may be helpful but it is not a key component of a phlebotomist's job requirements.

18.

A. Oncology is the department involved in the diagnosis and treatment of malignant (life-threatening) tumors. (p. 5)

B. Rheumatology is the department involved in the diagnosis and treatment of joint and tissue diseases, including arthritis.

C. Geriatrics is the department involved in the diagnosis and treatment of the elderly population.

D. Proctology is the department involved in the diagnosis and treatment of diseases of the anus and rectum.

19.

A. Phlebotomists do not routinely work with federal employees unless they are employed in a governmental hospital.

B. Phlebotomists must work with all other members of a health care team, not just laboratory personnel.

C. Phlebotomists must work with all other members of a health care team. (p. 11)

D. Phlebotomists must work with all members of a health care team, not just physicians.

20.

A. The neurology department deals with disorders and diseases of the nervous system.

B. The department of otolaryngology deals with disorders and diseases of the ears, nose, and throat.

C. The department of gastroenterology deals with diseases and disorders related to the esophagus, stomach, and intestines. (p. 4)

D. The department of endocrinology deals with disorders and diseases of the organs and tissues that produce hormones.

21.

A. The department of neurology deals with disorders and diseases of the nervous system.

B. The pulmonary division deals with disorders and diseases of the lungs.

C. The nephrology department deals with disorders and diseases of the kidneys. (p. 4)

D. Immunology is the department that deals with disorders and diseases of the immune system.

22.

A. Communication is a vital part of a phlebotomist's job role and does help improve "public opinion"; however, there are other reasons that are more important for having positive communication skills.

B. Positive communication can be good for business," but it is not the most important reason for good communication.

C. Positive communication for phlebotomists does not relate to Medicaid eligibility.

D. It is important for phlebotomists to take pleasure in communicating with patients because it improves the likelihood that the collection process will be successful. (p. 11)

23.

A. Radiotherapy departments relate to using high-energy x-rays in the treatment of diseases, particularly cancer.

B. Laboratory departments do not have emergency rooms.

C. Typical laboratory departments have two components, clinical pathology and surgical or anatomic pathology. (p. 12)

D. "Pharmacy testing" is not a phrase used in the laboratory.

24.

A. Ambulatory care refers to personal health care provided to an individual who is not bedridden.

B. Ambulatory care refers to personal health care provided to an individual who is not bedridden and therefore is an outpatient. (p. 3)

C. Ambulatory care refers to personal health care provided to an individual who is not bedridden.

D. Ambulatory care refers to personal health care provided to an individual who is not bedridden.

25.

A. Monitoring of the patient's health status through laboratory analysis is used to assure that the therapy or treatment is working to alleviate the medical condition.

B. Monitoring of the patient's health status to develop a community needs assessment can be very helpful to the overall community but sometimes does *not* fit the immediate monitoring needs on a particular patient. (p. 2)

C. Clinical laboratory technicians and clinical laboratory scientists perform tests, record laboratory procedures, and report results.

D. Therapeutic assessment through laboratory analysis are used to develop the appropriate therapy of treatment of the medical condition for the patient.

26.

A. Clinical laboratory scientists perform the microscopic analysis of blood smears, whereas the phlebotomist collects the blood smears for the microscopic analysis.

B. Clinical laboratory scientists participate in the development of new laboratory testing instrumentation; however, phlebotomists are not routinely involved in development of instrumentation.

C. Clinical laboratory technicians and clinical laboratory scientists perform tests and record immunologic laboratory procedures. Phlebotomists do not routinely test and record immunologic lab results.

D. The phlebotomist is involved in selecting and performing the appropriate quality control procedures such as monitoring the expiration dates on blood collection vacuum tubes. (pp. 6, 9–10)

27.

A. "Preassessment" is not a term used to define a phase of laboratory testing.

B. Phlebotomists play a vital role in the preanalytic phase of specimen collection, the part of the process that occurs before the actual testing and analysis is performed. The preanalytic process is the fundamental and crucial domain of every phlebotomist. (p. 12)

C. The analytical phase refers to the testing phase and fits into responsibilities of laboratory scientists and technicians.

D. The post-analytical phase refers to what happens after the actual testing takes place, that is, results are reported and follow-up documentation may be necessary.

28.

A. The federal government regulates all clinical laboratories through the Clinical Laboratory Improvement Amendments of 1988 (CLIA 1988). (p. 12)

B. The American Association of Blood Banks (AABB) has oversight only of clinical laboratories that have blood banking (transfusion medicine testing).

C. Medicaid, a federal and state program covering health services for the poor and other special populations, has oversight only of clinical laboratories that participate in Medicaid reimbursement.

D. Medicare, a federal program covering health services for the elderly, has oversight only of clinical laboratories that participate in Medicare reimbursement.

29.

A. Moving the patient to a different position for comfort is a positive behavior but may not relate to building rapport.

B. Building "rapport" involves developing a comfortable bond between the patient and the phlebotomist and involves common courtesy, showing interest in the patient, and building trust so as to improve communication and patient satisfaction. (p. 15)

C. Providing feedback about the patient's illness is not the phlebotomist's responsibility and should be left to the patient's physician.

D. Filing laboratory reports may indeed be a part of a phlebotomist's duties, but it does not relate to building rapport.

30.

A. As a courteous gesture, the patient should be asked if they mind reducing the volume or turning it off completely prior to performing the procedure. If a phlebotomist just turns it off without asking, it is rude and interrupts needlessly.

B. As a courteous gesture, the patient should be asked if they mind reducing the volume, using the mute function, or turning it off completely prior to performing the procedure. (p. 17)

C. The television can be a harmful distraction by preventing the patient from hearing the instructions about the procedure if it is too loud. In most cases, simply lowering the volume will alleviate the negative distraction (noise), yet allow the patient to have something to look at while enduring the procedure.

D. The patient's wishes should be the determining factor about whether or not the family members may stay in the room during the procedure and the phlebotomist should be courteous and respectful to them at all times.

31.

A. In some states, children are not permitted to serve as translators for their parents when health care issues are discussed.

B. In some states, children are not permitted to serve as translators for their parents when health care issues are discussed.

C. In some states, children are not permitted to serve as translators for their parents when health care issues are discussed. Phlebotomists should be knowledgeable of the applicable laws and their organization's policies and practices regarding translations. In many larger organizations, there are personnel available to assist with translations; additionally, online translation services and/or written instructions in languages other than English can be made available. (pp. 17–18)

D. Regardless of the language, the patient and family members should be spoken to in a respectful, articulate, and professional manner.

32.

A. Eye diseases and disorders are treated in the ophthalmology department.

B. The otolaryngology department is involved in the diagnosis and treatment of disorders and diseases related to the ears, nose, and throat. (pp. 4–5)

C. Bone and joint diseases and disorders are treated in the orthopedics department.

D. Skin diseases and disorders are treated in the dermatology department.

33.

A. This answer is inappropriate because the procedure does hurt.

B. This answer is inappropriate because the procedure usually hurts for more than one second.

C. This is a truthful and accurate answer and demonstrates to the patient that it is only a temporary discomfort. (p. 20)

D. While the procedure can be very uncomfortable for some patients, this statement instills undue fear and anxiety. Most patients only experience mild, temporary discomfort.

34.

A. The blood collector should state that the patient's physician ordered blood to be collected for testing and that it would be best to discuss the laboratory test with the physician. It is beyond the phlebotomist's scope of practice to discuss test results.

B. The blood collector should state that the patient's physician ordered blood to be collected for testing and that it would be best to discuss the laboratory test with the physician. Phlebotomists should be truthful about their "student" status.

C. The blood collector should state that the patient's physician ordered blood to be collected for testing and that it would be best to discuss the laboratory test with the physician. Again, it is beyond the phlebotomist's scope of practice to discuss or interpret laboratory results.

D. The blood collector should state that the patient's physician ordered blood to be collected for testing and that it would be best to discuss the laboratory test with the physician. (pp. 6, 10–11)

35.

A. The neonatology department treats and supports the needs of newborn and prematurely born babies. (pp. 4–5)

B. The neonatology department treats and supports the needs of newborn and prematurely born babies. Children who are 3–5 years old are "toddlers."

C. The neonatology department treats and supports the needs of newborn and prematurely born babies.

D. The neonatology department treats and supports the needs of newborn and prematurely born babies, not necessarily the mothers.

36.

A. Occupational therapists work in rehabilitation centers or hospitals to improve the functional abilities of patients. They do not have specimen collection duties.

B. The medical laboratory technician or clinical laboratory technician is typically an individual with a 2-year degree that performs designated laboratory testing, processing, and collecting of specimens. (p. 14)

C. Clinical laboratory scientists or medical technologists perform laboratory tests and operate sophisticated instruments for testing patients' specimens. They usually have a 4-year degree.

D. Physical therapists assist patients in restoring physical abilities that have been impaired by illness or injury. However, they do not have specimen collection duties.

37.

A. A bone marrow evaluation is a high-complexity test because it can lead to a reasonable risk of harm to the patient if results are inaccurate.

B. Urine cultures are categorized as a moderate-complexity test owing to the risk to the patient if results are inaccurate.

C. Waivered tests are those tests that are easiest to perform and least risky to patients. They include urinalysis. (p. 15)

D. Cytogenetics is in the category of high-complexity testing because it can lead to a reasonable risk of harm to the patient if results are inaccurate.

38.

A. When a stranger gets too close, it can cause the patient to feel nervous, fearful, or anxious. The phlebotomist should have slowed down, gently awakened the patient, then calmly explained the purpose for interrupting her sleep. The phlebotomist intruded the patient's zone of comfort and did so too quickly. (p. 24)

B. There was no indication that this patient was overmedicated.

C. The phlebotomist was in too much of a hurry for the patient to feel comfortable with the procedure. A slower, more professional approach to the patient would have enabled the patient to wake up and adjust to the situation.

D. There was no indication that the phlebotomist was overly cheerful and happy. In fact, if the phlebotomist had been more cautious about professional behavior, the encounter might have ended more positively.

39.

A, B, C. Culture encompasses values, beliefs, traditions, and practices of a group of individuals. It is important that health care workers demonstrate cultural sensitivity toward patients with cultural differences from their own.

D. Skin sensitivity is important, but not part of "cultural" sensitivity. (p. 25)

40.

A, B, C. In a health care setting, anyone involved in the health care process inside of the organization is a potential customer. This includes patients, family members, support groups, and all health care workers.

D. In a health care setting, anyone involved in the health care process inside of the organization is a potential customer. This includes patients, family members, support groups, and all health care workers. Special interest groups may be considered "external" stake holders, for example, advocacy groups (AARP), insurance companies, agencies that provide funding. (pp. 31–32)

41.

A. The phlebotomist should avoid making deep sighs around patients, since this can convey a feeling of being bored. (pp. 26–27)

B. A smile should *not* be avoided, since it makes the patient feel important.

C. Making eye contact with the patient should *not* be avoided. It conveys a sense of trust.

D. Maintaining relaxed hands, arms, and shoulders during blood collection shows that the phlebotomist has confidence and reassurance in his or her responsibilities.

42.

A. Geriatrics is the department that is specifically responsible for the diagnosis and treatment of the elderly population. (p. 4)

B. Internal medicine is a health care facility department that is involved in the general diagnosis and treatment of patients for problems of one or more internal organs.

C. Psychiatry/neurology is the department that is involved in the diagnosis and treatment for people of all ages with mental, emotional, and nervous system problems.

D. Proctology is the department in the health care facility that is involved in the diagnosis and treatment of diseases of the anus and rectum.

43.

A. Synovial fluid is analyzed in the clinical pathology area rather than the anatomic pathology area.

B. In the anatomic pathology area, autopsies are performed and surgical biopsy tissues are analyzed. (p. 13)

C. Cerebrospinal fluid (CSF) is analyzed in the clinical pathology area and sometimes in the anatomic pathology area.

D. Sputum fluid is analyzed in the clinical pathology area rather than the anatomic pathology area.

44.

A. Cytogenetics analysis and electrophoresis testing fall in the category of high-complexity tests, and they are not waivered.

B. Cytogenetics analysis and electrophoresis testing fall in the category of high-complexity tests. The term "extremely" high complexity is not used.

C. Cytogenetics analysis and electrophoresis testing fall in the category of high-complexity tests, since they are complex to perform and may allow for reasonable risk of harm to the patient if results are inaccurate. (p. 15)

D. Cytogenetics analysis and electrophoresis testing fall in the category of high-complexity tests, not moderate.

45.

A. The PDCA cycle does not represent a quality model for performing venipunctures.

B. The PDCA cycle represents a strategy for quality improvement. It uses a cycle of *planning* the change, *doing* the improvement, *collecting* the data and analyzing the results, *checking* the results to see whether the change improved the situation, and *acting* on what was learned by either rejecting the change, adjusting the change, or adopting the change as a standard part of the process. (p. 33)

C. The PDCA cycle does not represent a modified laboratory model.

D. The PDCA cycle does not represent a ten-step process for laboratory testing.

46.

A. Brainstorming is a technique to stimulate creative ideas.

B. Flowcharts break out components into a diagram for easier visualization of the process.

C. Pareto charts are bar charts that show the frequency of problems.

D. Cause-and-effect diagrams can be used in quality improvement methodologies and are designed to assist in identifying interactions between people, methods, equipment, and supplies. (p. 33)

47.

A. Pareto charts can be used in quality improvement methodologies to show the frequency of problematic events. The Pareto principle suggests that 80% of the trouble comes from 20% of the problems. (pp. 33, 35)

B. Brainstorming is a technique to stimulate creative ideas.

C. Cause-and-effect diagrams identify interactions between people, methods, equipment, and supplies.

D. Flowcharts break out components into a diagram for easier visualization of the process.

48.

A. Flowcharts can be used in quality improvement to break out components into a diagram for easier visualization and understanding of a process. (pp. 33–34)

B. Pareto charts are bar charts that show the frequency of problems.

C. Brainstorming is a technique to stimulate creative ideas.

D. Cause-and-effect diagrams identify interactions between people, methods, equipment, and supplies.

49.

A, B, C. Quality improvement efforts for specimen collection frequently involve assessment of the phlebotomist's technique, frequency of hematomas, recollection rates, and/or multiple sticks on the same patient.

D. Quality improvement efforts for specimen collection frequently involve assessment of the phlebotomist's technique, frequency of hematomas, recollection rates, and/or multiple sticks on the same patient. Drug reactions, while important, are normally beyond the phlebotomist's scope of practice. (pp. 36–38)

50.

A. Nosocomial infection rates are an example of outcomes that can be assessed for quality improvement purposes. (p. 32)

B. The presence of a pathologist 24 hours per day is an assessment of the management structure of the facility and also has less effect on the patient outcome unless there is a problem with a laboratory specimen or result.

C. The number of fire extinguishers available would be an assessment of the physical facility. While this is an important element, it has less effect on patient outcomes unless there is a fire in the facility.

D. "All of the above" is incorrect.

2 Ethical, Legal, and Regulatory Issues

chapter objectives

Upon completion of Chapter 2, the learner is responsible for the following:

- Define basic ethical and legal terms and explain how they differ.
- Describe the basic functions of the medical record.
- Define **informed consent.**
- Describe how to avoid litigation as it relates to blood collection.
- Identify key elements of the Health Insurance Portability and Accountability Act (HIPAA).

DIRECTIONS
Each of the questions or incomplete statements below is followed by four suggested answers or completions. Select one answer that is best in each case.

1. The best definition for ethics is:
   A. societal rules or regulations
   B. moral standards of behavior
   C. societal protection of the public
   D. conflict resolution through regulations

2. To evaluate an ethical decision, the health care worker should ask oneself ALL the following EXCEPT:
   A. Can I live with myself after making this decision?
   B. Is this legal and does it comply with institutional policy?
   C. Does it foster a "win–win" situation with the patient/supervisor or other individual?
   D. Can I avoid giving testimony at a trial?

3. Bioethics refer to:
   A. societal rules or regulations
   B. "life-and-death" issues
   C. moral standards of behavior
   D. protecting the welfare and safety of society

4. The legislative written laws are:
   A. made at the federal level only
   B. statutes made for the state level only
   C. statutes
   D. case law based on legal cases

5. The judicial branch of the government:
   A. provides statutes for society
   B. establishes case law
   C. provides administrative laws based on legal cases

D. uses legal cases to establish written statutes

6. Malpractice phlebotomy cases lead to decisions primarily made in what branch of government?
   A. legislative branch
   B. executive branch
   C. judicial branch
   D. state's legislative branch

7. When "a patient should be allowed to die" is a topic closely related to:
   A. the executive branch of the government
   B. moral issues of "bioethics"
   C. assault and battery
   D. civil law

8. A phlebotomist who just realized he has made a mistake in identifying a patient should first consider ALL of the following "ethics check" questions EXCEPT:
   A. Can I avoid giving testimony at a trial?
   B. Is this legal and does it comply with institutional policy?
   C. Does it foster a "win–win" situation with the patient/supervisor or other individual?
   D. Can I live with myself after making this decision?

9. In alleged negligence cases when "the plaintiff must be able to show what actually happened and that the defendant acted unreasonably," what factor does this indicate?
   A. breach of duty
   B. proximate causation

C. damages

D. duty

10. Misidentifying the patient, which can lead to confusion of patients' samples and possible wrong diagnosis and death, is considered:

A. assault

B. negligence

C. battery

D. a subpoena

11. An assault that is permissible is:

A. considered a breach of duty

B. malpractice

C. consent to obtain a blood specimen

D. a misdemeanor

12. If a phlebotomist gives his or her friend the results of a patient's drug abuse test results, what can be claimed by the patient against the phlebotomist?

A. assault

B. battery

C. negligence

D. misdemeanor

13. A patient claimed in court that the phlebotomist did not perform proper blood collection procedure that led to an alleged injury. The patient must show that the phlebotomist failed to meet:

A. the criminal laws in the state

B. the prevailing standard of care

C. the administrative laws of the state

D. HIPAA requirements

14. For a phlebotomist to collect blood for a research study in the health care institution, he or she must obtain consent from the research participant due to:

A. standard of care

B. IRB requirements

C. the American Hospital Association

D. CLIA

15. In past research studies, the unethical treatment of humans led to:

A. CLIA

B. HIPAA

C. The National Research Act

D. The Health Insurance Portability and Accountability Act

16. Which of the following organizations is influential in setting the "standard of care" for phlebotomy practice?

A. EPA

B. IRB

C. JCAHO

D. HIPAA

17. An IRB requires:

A. implied consent of the research participant

B. a blood collector in a research project to attend a course on the protection of the research participant

C. a statute of limitations

D. interpreters be present for the implied consent

18. In HIV-related issues for phlebotomists, the

A. employee is legally responsible for monitoring HIV post-exposure follow-up

B. incident report at the health care facility is not usually involved in legal issues

C. employer is legally responsible for monitoring HIV post-exposure follow-up

D. phlebotomist contracting AIDS during work will not be covered for health care if he or she discontinues work

19. The CLIA '88 was passed to:
    A. provide malpractice insurance coverage for laboratory personnel, including phlebotomists
    B. ensure the quality and accuracy of nursing care in health care facilities
    C. ensure the quality and accuracy of laboratory testing
    D. ensure that HIV testing occurred on all laboratory personnel

20. A phlebotomist performing which of the following procedures is considered a "CLIA-waived" procedure?
    A. venipuncture for a cross-match
    B. dipstick urinalysis
    C. skin puncture for a CBC
    D. venipuncture of a toxicology panel

21. If a phlebotomist makes a statement that is false regarding a patient, his action is:
    A. respondeat superior
    B. breach of duty
    C. malice
    D. a battery

22. If the phlebotomist has a lawsuit filed against him, he is the
    A. plaintiff
    B. defendant
    C. respondeat superior
    D. prosecutor

23. If the phlebotomist unintentionally hit the patient's median nerve in the venipuncture procedure, he or she
    A. is a felon
    B. has committed a crime
    C. can be accused of professional negligence
    D. will be handed a misdemeanor charge

24. Violation of patient confidentiality
    A. is considered respondeat superior
    B. is only considered in CLIA's moderately complex procedures
    C. can be considered professional negligence
    D. can be considered assault

25. The phrase "if you do not let me collect your blood, your infection will probably become severe" spoken by a phlebotomist to a patient can:
    A. lead to false imprisonment
    B. lead to an assault and battery charge
    C. create a situation where the phlebotomist becomes a plaintiff against the patient
    D. create a lawsuit under the HIPAA regulations

26. Which federal agency or Act states that a laboratory with moderately complex or highly complex testing must have written policies and procedures for specimen collection and labeling?
    A. FDA
    B. HCFA
    C. EPA
    D. CLIA

27. Before a patient's laboratory test results can legally be released, the patient must:
    A. express verbal permission
    B. tell his or her physician that it is okay
    C. provide written consent
    D. provide his or her lawyer's consent

28. The legal term for improper or unskillful care of a patient by a member of the health care team or any professional misconduct,

unreasonable lack of skill, or infidelity in professional or judiciary duties is:

A. malpractice

B. misdemeanor

C. litigation

D. liability

29. Which of the following legal branches writes regulations that enforce the laws?

A. administrative branch

B. judicial branch

C. U.S. Supreme Court

D. executive branch

30. One agency affecting regulations on blood collection is JCAHO. The abbreviation stands for:

A. Joint Care Administration and Hospital Organizations

B. Jurisprudence Care Administration and Hospital Organizations

C. Joint Commission on Accreditation of Healthcare Organizations

D. Jurisprudence Commission for Accreditation of Healthcare Organizations

31. The avoidance of legal conflicts in blood collection through education and planning is considered:

A. administrative law

B. executive law

C. preventive law

D. preparatory law

32. When should incident reports involving accidental HIV exposures be reported?

A. at the end of the work shift

B. immediately

C. after 24 hours

D. after seeing the employee health physician

33. Cross-examination is:

A. part of the HIPAA Act

B. used immediately when a malpractice lawsuit is filed

C. used during the trial to obtain information regarding the possibility of malpractice of a health care worker or in other types of trials as well

D. the same as a deposition

34. Mrs. Harriott, a phlebotomist who collects blood in Valley View Hospital from 6:00 A.M. to 12:00 P.M. during the week, recently suffered a needle puncture wound when a HIV-positive psychiatric patient from whom she was collecting blood kicked her. Valley View Hospital must report this accidental exposure incident to the:

A. FDA

B. EPA

C. CDC

D. OSHA

35. Examination of witnesses before and/or during a trial is referred to as:

A. discovery

B. statute of limitation

C. respondent superior

D. implied consent

36. All of the following are ways to avoid malpractice litigation *except:*

A. regularly participating in continuing education programs

B. reporting incidents within 48 hours

C. properly handling all confidential communications without violation

D. obtaining consent for collection of specimens

37. A nonmedical reason for using medical records from a patient is to:
    A. allow continuity of the patients' care plan
    B. allow for the health care institution's utilization review
    C. provide documentation of the patients' illness and treatment
    D. document communication between the physician and the health care team

38. The largest area of litigation regarding health care workers (including phlebotomists) is the:
    A. statute of limitations
    B. implied consent principle
    C. informed consent principle
    D. FDA requirements

39. Which of the following is the best example of setting the standard of care for blood collection?
    A. Texas Association of Clinical Laboratory Sciences
    B. Southwest Regional Phlebotomists' Association
    C. California Clinical Laboratory Association
    D. American Hospital Association

40. Professional negligence in blood collection is the same as:
    A. malice
    B. malpractice
    C. informed consent
    D. implied consent

41. When a health care provider gives aid at an accident, he or she is usually protected through:
    A. informed consent
    B. implied consent

C. CLIA 88
D. rightful action consent

42. Failure to act or perform duties according to standards of the profession is:
    A. battery
    B. negligence
    C. criminal action
    D. slander

43. Which of the following agencies requires an inspection for quality laboratory testing?
    A. FDA
    B. EPA
    C. OSHA
    D. CLIA

44. Which of the following maintains surveillance of health care workers' accident exposures?
    A. FDA
    B. JCAHO
    C. OSHA
    D. employers

45. In legal cases, "what a reasonably prudent person would do under similar circumstances" refers to:
    A. discovery
    B. standard of care
    C. informed consent
    D. implied consent

46. During a patient's appointment with his physician, he fills out the necessary legal papers and meets with his physician. After his physical exam, the physician orders laboratory tests for diagnosis and the patient comes to the laboratory with a rolled-up sleeve. The patient is giving:
    A. implied consent
    B. informed consent

C. rightful action consent

D. preventive consent

47. A child who refused to have his blood collected was locked in a room by a health care worker and was forced to have his blood collected. This is an example of:

A. informed consent

B. invasion of privacy

C. assault and battery

D. a misdemeanor

48. The standard of care currently used in phlebotomy malpractice legal cases involving health care providers is based on the conduct of the average health care provider in which area?

A. city

B. state

C. national community

D. regional community

49. Which legal concept refers to the voluntary permission by a patient to allow touching, examination, and/or treatment by health care providers?

A. implied consent

B. battery

C. informed consent

D. assault and battery

50. The law enacted in 1992 that regulates the quality and accuracy of laboratory testing (including blood collection) by creating a uniform set of provisions governing all clinical laboratories is referred to as:

A. CLIA 88

B. HCFA

C. FDA

D. EPA

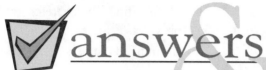

1.

A. Societal rules or regulations refer to laws.

B. Ethics are the moral standards of behavior. (p. 44)

C. Societal protection of the public comes from the laws instituted for the society.

D. Conflict resolution through regulations refers to the laws that regulate the public.

2.

A. Can I live with myself after making this decision? This is an ethical question.

B. Is this legal and does it comply with institutional policy? This is an ethical question to consider.

C. Does it foster a "win–win" situation with the patient/supervisor or other individual? This is an ethical question.

D. Can I avoid giving testimony at a trial? This is a legal question, not an ethical check. (p. 44)

3.

A. Societal rules or regulations refer to laws.

B. Bioethics refer to "life-and-death" issues. (p. 44)

C. Ethics are the moral standards of behavior.

D. Laws are the protection of the welfare and safety of society.

4.

A. Legislative written laws are statutes made at the federal, state, and county levels.

B. Legislative written laws are statutes made at the federal, state, and county levels.

C. Legislative written laws are statutes. (p. 44)

D. Legislative written laws are statutes.

5.

A. The judicial branch of the government establishes case law based on legal cases.

B. The judicial branch of the government establishes case law based on legal cases. (p. 44)

C. The judicial branch of the government establishes case law based on legal cases.

D. The judicial branch of the government establishes case law based on legal cases.

6.

A. Malpractice phlebotomy cases lead to decisions primarily made in the state and/or federal judicial branch.

B. Malpractice phlebotomy cases lead to decisions primarily made in the state and/or federal judicial branch.

C. Malpractice phlebotomy cases lead to decisions primarily made in the state and/or federal judicial branch. (pp. 54–55)

D. Malpractice phlebotomy cases lead to decisions primarily made in the state and/or federal judicial branch.

7.

A. Bioethics are moral issues or problems that refer to "life-and-death" issues such as abortion, when a patient should be allowed to die, etc.

B. Bioethics are moral issues or problems that refer to "life-and-death" issues such as abortion, when a patient should be allowed to die, etc. (p. 44)

C. Assault and battery is the intentional touching of another person without consent and carrying out of threatened physical harm.

D. Civil law involves suing for monetary damages.

8.

A. Can I avoid giving testimony at a trial? This question should _not_ be among the first to consider after misidentifying a patient. (p. 44)

B. Is this legal and does it comply with institutional policy? This question should be part of the "ethics check."

C. Does it foster a "win–win" situation with the patient/supervisor or other individual? This question should be part of the "ethics check."

D. Can I live with myself after making this decision? This question should be part of the "ethics check."

9.

A. Four factors must be considered in alleged negligence cases and the second one, breach of duty, indicates that "the plaintiff must be able to show what actually happened and that the defendant acted unreasonably." (p. 45)

B, C, D. Four factors must be considered in alleged negligence cases and the second one, breach of duty, indicates that "the plaintiff must be able to show what actually happened and that the defendant acted unreasonably."

10.

A. Assault is the unjustifiable attempt to touch another person or threat to do so.

B. Negligence is the failure to act or perform duties according to the standards of the profession that occurred in this example. Misidentification of a patient sample can be considered negligence. (p. 46)

C. Battery is the intentional touching of another person without consent.

D. A subpoena is a court order for a person and documents to be brought to court proceedings.

11.

A. A breach of duty is not permissible.

B. Malpractice is negligence in the health care field and is not considered permissible.

C. An assault is ONLY permissible if proper consent has been given such as consent to obtain a blood specimen. (p. 46)

D. A misdemeanor is a general term for all types of criminal offenses that are NOT permissible.

12.

A. Assault is the unjustifiable attempt to touch another person or threat to do so.

B. Battery is the intentional touching of another person without consent.

C. Negligence can be claimed if employees' or patients' drug abuse tests are released to anyone other than the attending physician or other authorized individual. (p. 47)

D. A misdemeanor is a criminal offense that is less serious than a felony.

13.

A, C, D. If a patient has suffered injury due to blood collection, the patient must show that the health care worker who collected the blood failed to meet the prevailing standard of care. These answers do not relate to the standard of care.

B. If a patient has suffered injury due to blood collection, the patient must show that the health care worker who collected the blood failed to meet the prevailing standard of care. (p. 47)

14.

A. Standards of care refer to the conduct and practice of the average health care worker. Standards of care are set by legal and regulatory entities.

B. The Institutional Research Boards (IRBs) at institutions (e.g., hospitals, universities) require that any research project utilizing human subjects require the informed consent of those subjects prior to their participation. (p. 48)

C, D. *Neither* the AHA or CLIA regulate blood collections for research purposes.

15.

A. The Clinical Laboratory Improvement Act (CLIA) was passed to ensure quality assurance in laboratory testing.

B. HIPAA was enacted to ensure confidentiality of patients' electronic medical records.

C. The unethical treatment of humans for research purposes led to the National Research Act. (p. 48)

D. The Health Insurance Portability and Accountability Act (HIPAA) was enacted to ensure confidentiality of patients' electronic medical records.

16.

A. EPA is the Environmental Protection Agency, which oversees environmental issues.

B. IRB refers to the "Institutional Research Boards," which oversees research activities.

C. JCAHO is the Joint Commission on Accreditation of Healthcare Organizations that is influential in setting the "standard of care." (pp. 47–48)

D. HIPAA is the federal law that requires maintenance of confidentiality of medical records.

17.

A. An IRB requires "informed consent," not "implied consent."

B. An IRB requires the blood collector in a research project to attend a course on the protection of research participants. (pp. 48–49)

C. Statute of limitations is a law that defines how soon after an injury due to malpractice that a plaintiff must file the lawsuit.

D. Interpreters are not usually required for implied consent.

18.

A. In HIV-related issues for phlebotomists, the employer is legally responsible for monitoring HIV post-exposure follow-up.

B. In HIV-related issues for phlebotomists, the incident report at the health care facility is very important to show a causal connection from patient to phlebotomist for the contraction of AIDS.

C. In HIV-related issues for phlebotomists, the employer is legally responsible for monitoring HIV post-exposure follow-up. (p. 47)

D. In HIV-related issues for phlebotomists, phlebotomists contracting AIDS during work-related activities will be covered for health care if he or she discontinues work.

19.

A. The CLIA '88 does not provide malpractice coverage.

B. The CLIA '88 does not cover issues related to nursing care.

C. The CLIA '88 was passed to ensure the quality and accuracy of laboratory testing. (p. 57)

D. The CLIA '88 does not ensure HIV testing for all laboratory personnel.

20.

A, C, D. Cross-matches, CBC's, and toxicology panels are *not* CLIA-waived tests.

B. A phlebotomist performing a dipstick urinalysis is considered CLIA waived. (p. 57)

21.

A. Respondeat superior is the concept whereby supervisors may be held liable for negligent actions of their employees.

B. Breach of duty refers to an infraction or failure to perform.

C. If a phlebotomist makes a statement that is false regarding a patient, this action is malice. (p. 46)

D. A battery refers to the intentional touching of another person without consent.

22.

A. If a phlebotomist has a lawsuit filed against him, he is the defendant, not the plaintiff.

B. If a phlebotomist has a lawsuit filed against him, he is the defendant. (p. 46)

C. Respondeat superior is the concept whereby supervisors may be held accountable for negligent actions of their employees.

D. If a phlebotomist has a lawsuit filed against him, he is the defendant, not the prosecutor.

23.

A, B, D. If the phlebotomist unintentionally hit the patient's median nerve during a venipuncture procedure, he or she can be accused of professional negligence. However, he or she is not automatically a felon, committed a crime, or been handed a misdemeanor charge.

C. If the phlebotomist unintentionally hit the patient's median nerve during a venipuncture procedure, he or she can be accused of professional negligence. (pp. 55–56)

24.

A. Violation of patient confidentiality can be considered professional negligence, not respondeat superior.

B. Violation of patient confidentiality can be considered professional negligence. It is not covered under CLIA

C. Violation of patient confidentiality can be considered professional negligence. (p. 47)

D. Violation of patient confidentiality can be considered professional negligence, not assault.

25.

A. The phrase "if you do not let me collect your blood, your infection will probably become severe" spoken by a phlebotomist to a patient can lead to an assault and battery charge.

B. The phrase "if you do not let me collect your blood, your infection will probably become severe" spoken by a phlebotomist to a patient can lead to an assault and battery charge. (p. 46)

C. The phrase "if you do not let me collect your blood, your infection will probably become severe" spoken by a phlebotomist to a patient can lead to an assault and battery charge.

D. The phrase "if you do not let me collect your blood, your infection will probably become severe" spoken by a phlebotomist to a patient can lead to an assault and battery charge.

26.

A. The Food and Drug Administration (FDA) evaluates the safety, clinical efficacy, and medical efficacy of the equipment and supplies used in blood collection.

B. The Health Care Financing Administration (HCFA) initially was the federal agency that required a laboratory with moderately complex or highly complex testing to have written policies and procedures for specimen collection and labeling.

C. The Environmental Protection Agency (EPA) monitors and enforces environmental requirements for the safe disposal of chemical and biological hazards.

D. The Clinical Laboratory Improvement Act (CLIA) is the act over clinical laboratory testing that has written policies and procedures for specimen collection and labeling. (p. 57)

27.

A. Before a patient's laboratory test results can legally be released, the patient must provide written consent, *not* just verbal permission.

B. Before a patient's laboratory test results can legally be released, the patient must provide written consent, not just a verbal "okay."

C. Before a patient's laboratory test results can legally be released, the patient must provide written consent. (p. 48)

D. Before a patient's laboratory test results can legally be released, the patient must provide written consent. It does not require a lawyer's consent.

28.

A. Malpractice is defined as improper or unskillful care of a patient by a member of the health care team or any professional misconduct or unreasonable lack of skill. (p. 46)

B. A misdemeanor is the general term for all sorts of criminal offenses that are not serious enough to be classified as felonies.

C. Litigation is the process of legal action to determine a decision in court.

D. Liability is the obligation to oversee damages.

29.

A. The executive branch writes regulations that enforce the laws.

B. The function of the judicial branch of the local, state, and federal government is to resolve disputes in accordance with the law.

C. The highest level within the judicial system is the U.S. Supreme Court. The function of the judicial branch is to resolve disputes in accordance with laws.

D. The executive branch writes regulations that enforce the laws. (p. 44)

30.

A. JCAHO stands for Joint Commission on Accreditation of Healthcare Organizations.

B. JCAHO stands for Joint Commission on Accreditation of Healthcare Organizations.

C. JCAHO stands for Joint Commission on Accreditation of Healthcare Organizations. (p. 48)

D. JCAHO stands for Joint Commission on Accreditation of Healthcare Organizations.

31.

A. Administrative law is the implementation of statutes and ordinances.

B. The avoidance of legal conflicts in blood collection through education and planning is called preventive law.

C. The avoidance of legal conflicts in blood collection through education and planning is called preventive law. (p. 52)

D. The avoidance of legal conflicts in blood collection through education and planning is called preventive law.

32.

A, C, D. An incident report involving accidental HIV exposure should be reported immediately. Actually, any blood collection incident needs to be reported immediately. These answers would cause unnecessary delays.

B. An incident report involving accidental HIV exposure should be reported immediately. Actually, any blood collection incident needs to be reported immediately. (p. 52)

33.

A. Cross-examination occurs at the trial that relates to the accusation of the malpractice that occurred by the health care worker. It is *not* part of HIPAA.

B. Cross-examination occurs at the trial that relates to the accusation of the malpractice that occurred by the health care worker. It is *not* used immediately when a lawsuit is filed.

C. Cross-examination occurs at the trial that relates to the accusation of the malpractice that occurred by the health care worker. (p. 50)

D. Cross-examination occurs at the trial that relates to the accusation of the malpractice that occurred by the health care worker. It is different from a deposition.

34.

A. The Food and Drug Administration (FDA) evaluates the safety, clinical efficacy, and medical efficacy of equipment and supplies in blood collection. It is not engaged in accidental exposure incidents.

B. The Environmental Protection Agency (EPA) monitors and enforces environmental requirements for the safe disposal of chemical and biological hazards. It is not engaged in accidental exposure incidents.

C. Employers are responsible for HIV postexposure follow-up testing. The health care institution must report accidental exposure incidents to the Centers for Disease Control and Prevention (CDC). (pp. 47, 128)

D. Employers are responsible for HIV post-exposure follow-up testing. The health care institution must report accidental exposure incidents to the Centers for Disease Control and Prevention (CDC).

35.

A. In legal terms, discovery is the right to examine the witness before the trial. (p. 50)

B. The statute of limitations defines time limits for filing lawsuits.

C. Respondeat superior is the concept whereby supervisors may be held liable for the actions of their employees.

D. Implied consent exists during an emergency when a patient's life is at risk and immediate action is required.

36.

A, C, D. To avoid malpractice litigation, it is extremely important to:

- obtain consent for collection of specimens
- regularly participate in continuing education programs
- report incidents immediately and document them
- properly handle all confidential communications without violation

B. To avoid malpractice litigation, it is extremely important to:

- **obtain consent for collection of specimens**
- **regularly participate in continuing education programs**
- **report incidents immediately (do *not* wait 48 hours) and document them**
- **properly handle all confidential communications without violation (pp. 52–53)**

37.

A, C, D. Documentation in the medical record about the patient's care plan, illness and treatment, or communication between the health care team are all medically-related reasons for using the medical record.

B. Medical records are sometimes used for nonmedical reasons that are not directly tied to

medical services, such as billing, utilization review, and quality improvement within the health care institution. (pp. 51–53)

38.

A. Health care workers are becoming more cognizant of the informed consent principle because this is the largest area of litigation.

B. Health care workers are becoming more cognizant of the informed consent principle because this is the largest area of litigation.

C. Health care workers are becoming more cognizant of the informed consent principle because this is the largest area of litigation. (p. 48)

D. Health care workers are becoming more cognizant of the informed consent principle because this is the largest area of litigation.

39.

A. All health care workers must conform to a specific standard of care to protect patients. In legal cases, the standard of care represents the conduct of the average health care worker in the community. The community has been expanded to the national community and is based on rules and regulations established by national professional organizations.

B. All health care workers must conform to a specific standard of care to protect patients. In legal cases, the standard of care represents the conduct of the average health care worker in the community. The community has been expanded to the national community and is based on rules and regulations established by national professional organizations.

C. All health care workers must conform to a specific standard of care to protect patients. In legal cases, the standard of care represents the conduct of the average health care worker in the community. The community has been expanded to the national community and is based on rules and regulations established by national professional organizations.

D. All health care workers must conform to a specific standard of care to protect patients. In legal cases, the standard of care represents the conduct of the average health care worker in the community. The community has been expanded to the national community and is based on rules and regulations established by national professional organizations. (pp. 47–48)

40.

A. Malice is related to making false statements.

B. Professional negligence is the improper or unskillful care of a patient by a member of the health care team and is usually referred to as malpractice. (p. 46)

C. Informed consent is voluntary permission by a patient to allow touching, examination, and/or treatment by health care providers.

D. Implied consent exists during an emergency when a patient's life is at risk and immediate action is required.

41.

A. Informed consent is voluntary permission by a patient to allow touching, examination, and/or treatment by health care providers.

B. Implied consent exists when immediate action is required to save a patient's life. (p. 49)

C. CLIA '88 is not involved in aid at an accident.

D. Informed consent is voluntary permission by a patient to allow touching, examination, and/or treatment by health care providers. The term "rightful action consent" is not used as a legal term.

42.

A. Battery is the intentional touching of another person without consent; it is also the unlawful beating of another or carrying out of threatened physical harm.

B. Failure to act or perform duties according to standards of the profession is negligence. (p. 46)

C. Criminal actions are legal recourse for acts or offenses against the public welfare.

D. Failure to act or perform duties according to standards of the profession is negligence.

43.

A, B, C. The FDA, EPA and OSHA do not require inspections except in special circumstances.

D. CLIA requires an inspection by federal and/or state agencies for quality laboratory testing. (p. 57)

44.

A. The Food and Drug Administration (FDA) evaluates the safety, clinical efficacy, and medical efficacy of the equipment and supplies used in blood collection.

B. The employers and Centers for Disease Control and Prevention (CDC) maintain national surveillance of health care workers' accidental exposure.

C. The employers and Centers for Disease Control and Prevention (CDC) maintain national surveillance of health care workers' accidental exposure.

D. The employers and Centers for Disease Control and Prevention (CDC) maintain national surveillance of health care workers' accidental exposure. (p. 53, 124)

45.

A. Discovery is to examine the witnesses before the trial to learn more regarding the nature and substance of each other's case.

B. In legal cases, the standard of care is determined by what a reasonably prudent person would do under similar circumstances. (pp. 47–48)

C. Informed consent is voluntary permission by a patient to allow touching, examination, and/or treatment by health care providers.

D. Implied consent exists when immediate action is required to save a patient's life or to prevent permanent impairment of the patient's health.

46.

A. Implied consent exists when immediate action is required to save a patient's life or to prevent permanent impairment of the patient's health.

B. Informed consent is voluntary permission by a patient to allow touching, examination, and/or treatment by health care providers. It allows patients to determine what will be performed on or to their bodies. By voluntarily rolling up his sleeve, the patient was allowing the health care provider to collect his blood. (p. 48)

C, D. Rightful action consent and preventive consent are not appropriate phrases.

47.

A. Informed consent is voluntary permission by a patient to allow touching, examination, and/or treatment by health care providers.

B. Invasion of privacy is the physical intrusion upon a person such as the publishing of confidential information.

C. Assault is the unjustifiable attempt to touch another person or threaten to do so in such circumstances as to cause the other to believe it will be carried out. Battery is the intentional touching of another person without consent and the unlawful beating of another or carrying out of the threatened physical harm (i.e., blood collection without consent). (p. 46)

D. A misdemeanor is a general term for all sorts of criminal offenses not serious enough to be classified as felonies.

48.

A, B, D. The standard of care currently used in phlebotomy malpractice legal cases and other health care malpractice legal cases is based on the national community as a result of national standards and requirements, *not* city, state, or regional areas.

C. The standard of care currently used in phlebotomy malpractice legal cases and other health care malpractice legal cases is based on the national community as a result of national standards and requirements. (pp. 47–48)

49.

A. Implied consent exists when immediate action is required to save a patient's life or to prevent permanent impairment of the patient's health.

B. Battery is the intentional touching of another person without consent.

C. Informed consent refers to the voluntary permission by a patient to allow touching, examination, and/or treatment by health care providers. (p. 48)

D. Assault is an unjustifiable attempt to touch another person, and battery is the intentional touching of another person without consent.

50.

A. In October 1988, the U.S. Congress passed the Clinical Laboratory Improvement Amendments (CLIA). The law is referred to as CLIA 88 and became effective in 1992 as a means to ensure the quality and accuracy of laboratory testing (including blood collection). (p. 57)

B. The Health Care Financing Administration (HCFA) is the federal agency that originally administered CLIA regulations.

C. The Food and Drug Administration (FDA) evaluates the safety, clinical efficacy, and medical efficacy of equipment and supplies used in blood collection.

D. The Environmental Protection Agency (EPA) monitors and enforces environmental requirements for the safe disposal of chemical and biological hazards.

answers & rationales

3 Basic Anatomy and Physiology of Organ Systems

chapter objectives

Upon completion of Chapter 3, the learner is responsible for the following:

➤ Define the terms *anatomy, physiology,* and *pathology.*

➤ Describe the directional terms, anatomic surface regions, and cavities of the body.

➤ Describe the role of homeostasis in normal body functioning.

➤ Describe the purpose, function, and structural components of the 11 body systems.

➤ Identify examples of disorders associated with each organ system.

➤ List common diagnostic tests associated with each organ system.

DIRECTIONS Each of the questions or incomplete statements below is followed by four suggested answers or completions. Select one answer that is best in each case.

1. The fact that the human body is bisymmetrical means which of the following?
   A. mouth and nose are both present
   B. it can be divided into halves that are alike
   C. hair serves to protect the skin
   D. organs are placed deep within the body for protection

2. Upper extremities include which regions of the body?
   A. ankle and foot
   B. leg
   C. arm and wrist
   D. pelvis

3. The human torso includes which of the following regions of the body?
   A. leg and foot
   B. arm and wrist
   C. face
   D. thorax and abdomen

4. Lungs are found in which of the following body cavities?
   A. cranial
   B. abdominopelvic
   C. thoracic
   D. spinal

5. The study of anatomy is best characterized by which of the following?
   A. functional components of the body
   B. biochemical makeup of the body
   C. anabolic and catabolic mechanisms in the body
   D. structural components of the body

6. Physiology is the study of:
   A. mechanical makeup of the body
   B. anabolic and catabolic mechanisms in the body
   C. functional components of the body
   D. structural components of the body

7. The anterior or ventral surface of the body has which of the following body cavities?
   A. abdominal only
   B. cranial
   C. spinal
   D. thoracic, abdominal, and pelvic

8. The posterior or dorsal surface is divided into which of the following cavities?
   A. thoracic, abdominal, and pelvic
   B. spinal only
   C. abdominal only
   D. cranial and spinal

9. The proximal end of the forearm means which of the following?
   A. near the elbow
   B. around the fingers
   C. near the wrist
   D. by the shoulder

10. When speaking with a patient about which arm to use for a venipuncture, how should a phlebotomist refer to the right or left one?

A. refer to the phlebotomist's right/left side

B. refer to the patient's right/left arm

C. face the same way the patient is facing and point to the arm

D. don't talk about it, just proceed with the arm that looks the best

11. The supine position refers to which of the following?

A. erect and standing

B. lying face-up on their back

C. lying face-down on their stomach

D. lying on the right side

12. Homeostasis refers to:

A. blood clotting

B. a chemical imbalance

C. an anabolism

D. the steady-state condition

13. Which of the following pairs are not opposite regions or planes of the body?

A. lateral/medial

B. distal/proximal

C. anterior/posterior

D. anterior/interior

For Questions 14–17, refer to Figure 3.1 and match the body plane or region shown in the figure with the one correct answer.

14. The body plane or region marked as "A" in Figure 3.1 represents which of the following?

A. sagittal

B. cranial/caudal

C. dorsal/ventral

D. transverse

FIGURE 3.1.

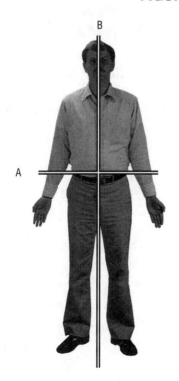
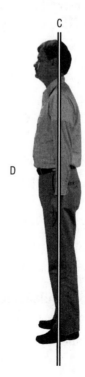

15. The body plane or region marked as "B" in Figure 3.1 represents which of the following?
    A. transverse
    B. sagittal
    C. dorsal/ventral
    D. cranial/caudal

16. The body plane or region marked as "C" in Figure 3.1 represents which of the following?
    A. ventral
    B. cranial/caudal
    C. transverse
    D. sagittal

17. The body region marked as "D" in Figure 3.1 represents which of the following?
    A. transverse
    B. sagittal
    C. cranial
    D. ventral

18. Which of the following body systems provide carbon dioxide and oxygen exchange?
    A. muscular
    B. respiratory
    C. reproductive
    D. nervous

19. Which of the following body systems is the primary regulator of hormones?
    A. digestive
    B. integumentary
    C. urinary
    D. endocrine

20. The pituitary gland is often referred to as:
    A. germ cells
    B. the "master gland"
    C. lymph tissue
    D. the respiratory control gland

21. How many chromosomes are contained in human cells?
    A. 46
    B. 50
    C. 25
    D. 100

22. What are vital signs?
    A. excess water in lungs
    B. overheated body temperature
    C. excessive respiration and pulse
    D. temperature, pulse, blood pressure, respiration rate

23. Meninges are defined as:
    A. control nerves
    B. causative agent of meningitis
    C. control reflexes
    D. protective membrane layers

24. Which organ secretes bile?
    A. stomach
    B. appendix
    C. pancreas
    D. liver

25. What are the primary components of the urinary system?
    A. kidneys
    B. hormones
    C. intestines
    D. cells in the liver

26. The endocrine system can best be evaluated by:
    A. tissue biopsy
    B. testing spinal fluid
    C. doing blood gas analyses
    D. analyzing hormone levels

27. Which structure governs the functions of the individual cell such as growth, repair, reproduction, and metabolism?
    A. lysosome
    B. cytoplasm
    C. nucleus
    D. membrane

28. Cell metabolism involves energy production by:
    A. breaking down chemical substances
    B. perspiration
    C. DNA transfer
    D. hemolysis

29. How many lobes do normal human lungs have?
    A. 2
    B. 3
    C. 5
    D. 4

30. The molecule that transports oxygen and carbon dioxide is:
    A. chloride
    B. alveoli
    C. hemoglobin
    D. carbon

31. After oxygen crosses the respiratory membranes (in the lung) into the blood, about 97% of it combines with:
    A. carbon dioxide
    B. the iron-containing portion of hemoglobin
    C. carbaminohemoglobin
    D. hypochloride

32. What is the blood pH range of a normal body?
    A. 7.5 to 8.0
    B. 7.35 to 7.45
    C. 0 to 7
    D. 6.5 to 10

33. Laboratory testing of the muscular system would include:
    A. creatine kinase and lactate dehydrogenase
    B. serum calcium
    C. urine culture
    D. synovial fluid

34. An XX pair of chromosomes means that the fetus will be:
    A. a baby boy
    B. a brown-haired child
    C. a baby girl
    D. a blue-eyed child

35. The skeletal system:
    A. provides pathways for nerve functions
    B. provides germ cell formation
    C. secretes hormones
    D. provides support, leverage, and movement

36. Functions of the skin include all but which one:
    A. secretion of oils
    B. prevention of water loss
    C. respiration
    D. production of perspiration

37. Which of the following body systems has the functions of communication, control, and integration?
    A. integumentary
    B. digestive
    C. nervous
    D. skeletal

38. Melanin is described as:
    A. a heat insulator
    B. a pigment that provides skin color
    C. a means of protecting tissues from infections
    D. a covering for the brain and spinal cord

39. Which of the following is a characteristic of DNA?
    A. contains thousands of genes
    B. is a double helix
    C. is located in the nucleus
    D. all of the above

40. Bones and cartilage compose the skeletal system. How does cartilage differ from bone?
    A. it is very porous
    B. it is rigid
    C. it allows for more flexibility
    D. it is calcified

41. Laboratory tests that evaluate the skeletal system include all but which one of the following?
    A. alkaline phosphatase
    B. follicle stimulating hormone
    C. synovial fluid analysis
    D. serum calcium

42. Disorders of the skeletal system include all but which one of the following?
    A. arthritis and bursitis
    B. gout
    C. bacterial infections
    D. hyperthyroidism

43. Which components make up the nervous system?
    A. blood cells and bone marrow
    B. neurons, brain, and spinal cord

C. cartilage coverings
D. fluid

44. Disorders of the nervous system include which of the following?
    A. amyotrophic lateral sclerosis
    B. Parkinson's disease
    C. encephalitis and meningitis
    D. all of the above

45. The creatinine clearance test evaluates which of the following?
    A. the kidneys' ability to filter out waste products
    B. red blood cell functioning
    C. white blood cell morphology
    D. abnormal respiration rate

46. All but which one of the following statements describes the lungs?
    A. contain branches of alveoli with surrounding capillaries
    B. release large amounts of carbon dioxide
    C. take in large amounts of oxygen
    D. produce hormones

47. In lung capillaries, the pressure of carbon dioxide decreases and the pressure of oxygen increases. This causes:
    A. hyperventilation
    B. oxygen to combine with hemoglobin
    C. formation of free oxygen molecules
    D. chemical combustion

48. The digestive system functions include:
    A. transporting oxygen and carbon dioxide
    B. breaking down food and eliminating waste
    C. secreting hormones for regulatory functions
    D. controlling nerve impulses

49. Disorders of the respiratory system include:
    A. ulcers
    B. melanoma
    C. polyps
    D. pneumonia, influenza, emphysema, and cystic fibrosis

50. Components of the lymphatic system include all but which one:
    A. bile duct
    B. tonsils
    C. lymph nodes
    D. bone marrow

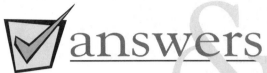

answers & rationales

1.

A. Mouth and nose do not relate to bisymmetry.

B. The term bisymmetry means that if an imaginary line (mid-sagittal plane) is drawn through the body in the middle, from front to back, both halves will be almost identical. (pp. 62, 65)

C. The hair does not relate to bisymmetry.

D. Organs are placed within the body for protection, however, it does not relate to bisymmetry.

2.

A and B. The ankle, foot, and leg are lower extremities.

C. The arm and wrist are upper extremities as are the shoulder, elbow, and hand regions. (p. 62)

D. The pelvis is generally considered part of the torso.

3.

A. The foot and leg are lower extremities.

B. The arm and wrist are upper extremities.

C. The face is considered part of the head region.

D. The thorax, abdomen, and pelvis are considered the torso. (p. 62)

4.

A. The cranial cavity holds the brain.

B. The abdominopelvic cavity holds the stomach, intestines, spleen, pancreas, liver, bladder, and reproductive organs.

C. The thoracic cavity holds the lungs. (pp. 63–64)

D. The spinal cavity holds the spinal cord.

5.

A. Physiology is the study of functional components of the body.

B. Physiology includes the study of the body's biochemical makeup.

C. Anabolic and catabolic mechanisms are reactions that produce energy and change complex substances into simpler ones, respectively.

D. Anatomy is the study of structural components of the body. (p. 62)

6.

A. Physiology is not the study of the mechanical makeup of the body.

B. Anabolic and catabolic mechanisms are important in metabolism.

C. Physiology is the study of the functional components of the body. (p. 62)

D. Anatomy is the study of structural components of the body.

7.

A. The anterior or ventral portions of the body contain other cavities in addition to the abdominal.

B. The cranial cavity is in the posterior or dorsal portion of the body.

C. The spinal cavity is in the posterior or dorsal portion of the body.

D. The anterior or ventral surface of the body has the thoracic, abdominal, and pelvic cavities. (pp. 63–65)

8.

A. The anterior or ventral surface contains the thoracic, abdominal, and pelvic cavities.

B. The posterior or dorsal portions of the body contain other cavities in addition to the spinal.

C. The posterior or dorsal portions of the body contain other cavities in addition to the abdominal.

D. The posterior or dorsal surface is divided into cranial and spinal cavities. (pp. 63–65)

9.

A. The proximal end of the forearm means near the elbow. (p. 66)

B. The area around the fingers is the distal end of the hand.

C. The area near the wrist is the distal end of the forearm.

D. The area by the shoulder is the proximal end of the arm.

10.

A. Phlebotomists should *not* refer to their own right and left sides when addressing the patient about which arm to use for venipuncture.

B. Phlebotomists should become accustomed to referring to the *patient's* right or left sides. It can be confusing when the phlebotomist is face-to-face with the patient. (p. 66)

C. This procedure is not necessary or appropriate.

D. This procedure is not appropriate.

11.

A. Erect standing position is the normal anatomic position.

B. The supine position is lying face-up on the back and is the best position for performing phlebotomy on patients who are bedridden. (p. 66)

C. The prone position is lying face-down on the stomach.

D. Lying on the right or left side is called the lateral recumbent position.

12.

A. Blood clotting is part of a process known as hemostasis.

B. Chemical imbalance is the opposite of a steady-state condition.

C. Anabolism refers to energy production by cells.

D. Homeostasis refers to a steady-state or chemically balanced condition in the body. (p. 65)

13.

A. Lateral/medial refers to opposite regions.

B. Distal/proximal refers to opposite regions.

C. Anterior/posterior refers to opposite regions.

D. Opposite regions or planes of the body are anterior/posterior, distal/proximal, and lateral/medial; anterior/interior are *not* opposite regions or body planes. (pp. 65–66)

For Questions 14–17, refer to Figure 3.1 and match the body plane or region shown in the figure with the one correct answer.

14.

A, B, C are incorrect answers.

D. The body plane/region marked as "A" in Figure 3.1 represents the transverse plane, which runs crosswise or horizontally, dividing the body into upper and lower sections. (pp. 63–65)

15.

A, C, D are incorrect answers.

B. The body plane marked as "B" in Figure 3.1 represents the sagittal plane, which runs lengthwise from front to back, dividing the body into right and left halves. (pp. 63–65)

16.

A, C, D are incorrect answers.

B. The body region marked as "C" in Figure 3.1 represents the cranial (close to the head) or superior (above) region. (pp. 63–65)

17.

A, B, C are incorrect answers.

D. The body region marked as "D" in Figure 3.1 represents the ventral (front side) or anterior (in front of) surface of the body. (pp. 63–65)

FIGURE 3.1. Body planes/regions.

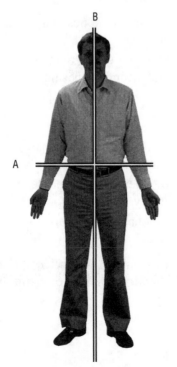
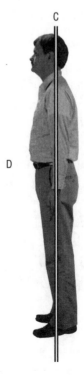

18.

A. The muscular system is responsible for movement.

B. The respiratory system is involved in carbon dioxide and oxygen exchange. (p. 78)

C. The reproductive system is responsible for birth.

D. The nervous system is responsible for control and communication.

19.

A. The reproductive system is responsible for birth.

B. The integumentary system is involved in the body's protection and regulation.

C. The urinary system produces and eliminates urine.

D. The endocrine system is the primary regulator of hormones. (pp. 83–84)

20.

A. Germ cells include ova and sperm.

B. The pituitary is often referred to as the "master gland" because it controls and regulates many functions of the body through hormone production. (p. 83)

C. Lymph tissue is a vague term referring to the lymphatic system, which is responsible for maintaining fluid balance in the tissues, providing defense against disease, and absorbing fats from digestion.

D. There is no such terminology as "respiratory control gland."

21.

A. Normal human cells contain 46 chromosomes. (p. 84)

B. There are not 50 chromosomes in a normal human cell.

C. There are not 25 chromosomes in a normal human cell.

D. There are not 100 chromosomes in a normal human cell.

22.

A. Excess water in the lungs is not a normal condition but does not involve all vital signs.

B. Increased body temperature would be an example of one vital sign only.

C. Respiration and pulse are examples of vital signs; however, it is not a complete answer.

D. Temperature, pulse, blood pressure, and respiration rate are considered vital signs. (p. 69)

23.

A. Meninges do not control nerves.

B. Meninges do not cause meningitis.

C. Meninges do not control reflexes.

D. Meninges are the protective membranes that cover the brain and spinal cord. Between these membranes is cerebrospinal fluid (CSF) that is also protective in nature. Phlebotomists are often responsible for transporting CSF to the laboratory for analysis. (p. 73)

24.

A. The stomach does not secrete bile; it secretes acid.

B. The appendix does not secrete bile or other substances.

C. The pancreas does not secrete bile; it manufactures and secretes insulin.

D. The liver secretes bile, which aids in fat digestion and absorption. This aids the body by helping to maintain homeostasis. (p. 79)

25.

A. Kidneys filter out water and solutes and re-absorb only the necessary amounts of these substances into the blood. Excess water and wastes are excreted as urine. (p. 81)

B. Hormones are produced in the endocrine system.

C. Intestines are part of the digestive system.

D. Cells in the liver secrete bile and are not part of the urinary system.

26.

A. Tissue biopsy would not reveal abnormalities in the endocrine system.

B. Spinal fluid analyses are useful for evaluating the nervous system.

C. Blood gas analyses are useful for evaluating the respiratory system.

D. Since the endocrine system regulates hormone production, laboratory analysis of hormone levels is one way to evaluate abnormalities in this body system. (pp. 83–84)

27.

A. The lysosome releases digestive enzymes for food digestion.

B. The cytoplasm contains organelles and is composed mostly of water.

C. The cell nucleus governs the functions of each individual cell. (p. 67)

D. The cell membrane is a protective barrier and allows substances to move in and out selectively.

28.

A. Metabolism involves making necessary substances or breaking down chemical substances to use energy. (p. 67)

B. Perspiration involves water loss from the skin.

C. Metabolism does not involve DNA transfer.

D. Hemolysis occurs when red blood cells rupture.

29.

A. Humans have two lungs with five lobes.

B. Humans have two lungs with five lobes.

C. Normal humans have two lungs. The left lung has only two lobes, and the right lung has three lobes. (p. 78)

D. Humans have two lungs with five lobes.

30.

A. Chloride is an electrolyte often evaluated in the laboratory.

B. Alveoli are grapelike structures in the lungs that allow diffusion of gases between air and blood.

C. Red blood cells transport gases as part of a molecule called hemoglobin. (p. 78)

D. Carbon is a building block of organic substances.

31.

A. Carbon dioxide does not combine with oxygen. It is exchanged for oxygen.

B. Oxygen combines with hemoglobin in the capillaries of the lungs. (p. 78)

C. Carbaminohemoglobin is a molecule containing hemoglobin and carbon dioxide.

D. Hypochloride does not combine with oxygen.

32.

A. The normal human blood pH range is not 7.5–8.0.

B. The normal blood pH of a human body has a narrow range of between 7.35 and 7.45. (p. 78)

C. The normal human blood pH range is not 0–7.

D. The normal human blood pH range is not 6.5–10.

33.

A. Laboratory testing of the muscular system could include assays of specific muscle enzymes such as creatine kinase and lactate dehydrogenase, analysis of autoimmune antibodies, microscopic examination, or culturing muscle tissue biopsies. (p. 73)

B. Serum calcium would be useful in assessing the skeletal system.

C. Urine culture would be useful for diagnosing a urinary tract infection.

D. Synovial fluid analysis would be useful in assessment of the joints.

34.

A. An XY pair of chromosomes would indicate a baby boy.

B. In this situation the hair color cannot be determined.

C. An XX pair of chromosomes indicates that the baby will be a girl. (p. 84)

D. In this situation the eye color cannot be determined.

35.

A. The nervous system provides pathways for nerve functions.

B. The reproductive system functions in germ cell formation.

C. The endocrine system is primarily responsible for secreting hormones.

D. The skeletal system provides bodily support and allows for leverage and movement. (pp. 70–72)

36.

A. Skin functions to secrete oils.

B. Skin functions to prevent water loss.

C. Skin prevents water loss and allows for perspiration as needed by the body during exercise, fever, or weather conditions. Skin does not function in respiration. (pp. 69–70)

D. Skin functions to produce perspiration.

37.

A. The integumentary system functions to regulate body temperature, receive sensory stimuli, and protect underlying tissues.

B. The digestive system functions in the breakdown of food.

C. Both the endocrine and the nervous systems function for communication, control, and integration of bodily functions. (pp. 73, 83)

D. The skeletal system provides support and movement and produces blood cells.

38.

A. Melanin does not act as a heat insulator.

B. Melanin provides skin color and protects underlying tissues from absorbing ultraviolet rays from the sun. (p. 69)

C. Melanin does not protect tissues from infections.

D. Meninges are coverings for the brain and spinal cord.

39.

A. DNA contains thousands of genes.

B. DNA is a double helix.

C. DNA is located in the nucleus.

D. DNA is described as a "double helix" or "twisted ladder." It is located in the nucleus and contains thousands of genes. It is not the same in all individuals, since it contains codes for the individual's genetic makeup. (p. 67)

40.

A. Bone, not cartilage, is a very porous material.

B. Bone, not cartilage, is rigid.

C. Cartilage is flexible and is surrounded by gelatinous material, in contrast to bone, which is calcified and rigid. (p. 70)

D. Bone, not cartilage, is calcified.

41.

A. Serum alkaline phosphatase is used to provide results for diagnostic and therapeutic monitoring.

B. Follicle stimulating hormone (FSH) is not used to evaluate the skeletal system. It is used in evaluating the reproductive system. (pp. 71, 85)

C. Synovial fluid analysis is used to provide results for diagnostic and therapeutic monitoring.

D. Serum calcium, is used to provide results for diagnostic and therapeutic monitoring.

42.

A. Arthritis and bursitis are disorders of the skeletal system.

B. Gout is a disorder of the skeletal system.

C. Bacterial infections also affect the skeletal system.

D. Disorders of the skeletal system include inflammatory conditions (arthritis and bursitis); gout; bacterial infections such as osteomyelitis; porous bone conditions such as osteoporosis; developmental conditions such as giantism, dwarfism, and rickets; and bone tumors. Hypo- and hyperthyroidism are disorders of the endocrine system. (pp. 71, 84)

43.

A. Blood cells and bone marrow are components of the cardiovascular system.

B. The nervous system is composed of specialized nerve cells (neurons), brain, spinal cord, brain and cord coverings, fluid, and the nerve impulse itself. (p. 73)

C. Cartilage is a component of the skeletal system.

D. The nervous system has cerebrospinal fluid but that is only a part of the system.

44.

A. Amyotrophic lateral sclerosis is a disorder of the nervous system.

B. Parkinson's disease is a disorder of the nervous system.

C. Encephalitis and meningitis are disorders of the nervous system.

D. Disorders of the nervous system include encephalitis, meningitis, tetanus, herpes, and poliomyelitis and conditions such as amyotrophic lateral sclerosis, multiple sclerosis, Parkinson's disease, cerebral palsy, tumors, epilepsy, hydrocephaly, neuralgia, and headaches. (pp. 73–75)

45.

A. The creatinine clearance test evaluates the degree to which kidneys are filtering out waste products of metabolism. (pp. 81–83)

B, C, D. The creatinine clearance does not evaluate red blood cell functioning, white blood cell morphology, or respiration rate.

46.

A. Lungs contain branches of alveoli with surrounding capillaries.

B. Lungs release large amounts of carbon dioxide.

C. Lungs take in large amounts of oxygen.

D. Lungs contain branches of alveoli surrounded by capillaries. They are able to take in large amounts of oxygen and release carbon dioxide. They are soft and spongy and reach from just above the collarbone to the diaphragm. Lungs do not produce hormones; the endocrine system produces hormones. (pp. 78, 83)

by body cells and, second, to eliminate the waste products of digestion. (pp. 79–80)

C. The digestive system does not secrete hormones for regulatory functions; the endocrine system does.

D. The nervous system controls and integrates nerve impulses.

47.

A. Hyperventilation does not result in normal respiration.

B. In lung capillaries, the pressure of oxygen increases and the pressure of carbon dioxide decreases, allowing oxygen to rapidly associate, or combine chemically, with hemoglobin at the same time that carbon dioxide dissociates, or is released, from carbaminohemoglobin. Thus in the lungs, humans inhale oxygen and exhale carbon dioxide. (p. 78)

C. Oxygen molecules are quickly combined with hemoglobin in the lung capillaries.

D. Chemical combustion does not occur in the lung capillaries.

48.

A. The respiratory and circulatory systems transport oxygen and carbon dioxide.

B. The digestive system functions, first, to break down food chemically and physically into nutrients that can be absorbed and used

---

49.

A. An ulcer is a disorder of the digestive system.

B. Melanoma is a type of skin cancer.

C. Polyps occur in the intestinal track.

D. Disorders of the respiratory system include tuberculosis, laryngitis, bronchitis, whooping cough, pneumonia, influenza, asthma, emphysema, cystic fibrosis, and tumors. (pp. 77–79)

50.

A. The lymphatic system includes the lymph nodes, tonsils, bone marrow, spleen, and thymus gland. The liver contains the bile duct. (pp. 85–86)

B. Tonsils are only one component of the lymphatic system.

C. Lymph nodes are only one component of the lymphatic system.

D. Bone marrow is only one component of the lymphatic system.

4 The Cardiovascular System

chapter objectives

Upon completion of Chapter 4, the learner is responsible for the following:

➤ Identify and describe the structures and functions of the heart.

➤ Trace the flow of blood through the cardiovascular system.

➤ Identify and describe the structures and functions of different types of blood vessels.

➤ Identify and describe the cellular and noncellular components of blood.

➤ Locate and name the veins most commonly used for phlebotomy procedures.

DIRECTIONS Each of the questions or incomplete statements below is followed by four suggested answers or completions. Select one answer that is best in each case.

1. Which of the following functions is *not* a function of the cardiovascular system?
   A. transportation of nerve impulses.
   B. transportation of water and nutrients
   C. transportation of gases
   D. coagulation process

2. The term "systole" refers to:
   A. capillary dialation
   B. heart contraction
   C. heart relaxation
   D. pulmonary gas exchange

3. The term "diastole" refers to:
   A. capillary dialation
   B. heart contraction
   C. heart relaxation
   D. pulmonary gas exchange

4. In what location of the body does oxygen and carbon dioxide gas exchange take place?
   A. alveoli of the lungs
   B. heart
   C. arteries
   D. veins

5. How many times does the average normal adult heart beat each minute?
   A. 15–20
   B. 25–30
   C. 40–60
   D. 60–80

6. The term "leukocytes" is another name for:
   A. red blood cells
   B. white blood cells
   C. platelets
   D. sera

7. The term "erythrocytes" is another name for:
   A. red blood cells
   B. white blood cells
   C. platelets
   D. sera

8. The term "thrombocytes" is another name for:
   A. red blood cells
   B. white blood cells
   C. platelets
   D. sera

9. Serum is the liquid portion of a blood sample that:
   A. is highly oxygenated
   B. contains anticoagulant
   C. does not contain anticoagulant
   D. is rich in carbon monoxide

10. A plasma specimen refers to blood that:
    A. is highly oxygenated
    B. contains fibrinogen
    C. does not contain anticoagulant
    D. is rich in carbon monoxide

11. Capillaries have which of the following characteristics?
    A. Transport deoxygenated blood toward the heart.
    B. Transport oxygenated blood away from the heart.
    C. Vessels linking arterioles and venules.
    D. They carry only white blood cells.

12. Arteries have which of the following characteristics?

    A. Transport deoxygenated blood toward the heart.

    B. Transport oxygenated blood away from the heart.

    C. Vessels linking arterioles and venules.

    D. They carry only red blood cells.

13. Veins have which of the following characteristics?

    A. Transport deoxygenated blood toward the heart.

    B. Transport oxygenated blood away from the heart.

    C. Vessels linking arterioles and venules.

    D. They carry only red blood cells.

14. Which of the following reflects the primary function of leukocytes?

    A. oxygen transport

    B. host cells

    C. blood clotting

    D. defense against infections

15. Which of the following reflects the primary function of erythrocytes?

    A. oxygen transport

    B. host cells

    C. blood clotting

    D. defense against infections

16. Which of the following reflects the primary function of platelets?

    A. oxygen transport

    B. host cells

    C. blood clotting

    D. defense against infections

17. The process of blood cell development (hematopoeisis) includes which of the following?

    A. Cells begin as undifferentiated stem cells.

    B. It occurs every 200 days.

    C. It occurs in the lungs.

    D. Requires large volumes of water.

18. Which of the following features does *not* characterize RBCs?

    A. biconcave disks that measure about 7 μm in diameter

    B. have no nuclei when circulating in the peripheral blood

    C. have a life span of about 120 days

    D. are smaller and more compact than platelets

19. The upper chambers of the heart are the:

    A. right and left atrium

    B. right and left ventricle

    C. inferior and superior vena cava

    D. reticulocytes

20. The four chambers of the heart include the:

    A. right and left atria and ventricles

    B. four sided ventricles

    C. four sided atria

    D. superior and inferior chambers

21. Which statement describes plasma?

    A. It results when cellular components form a fibrin clot.

    B. It is normally bright or fluorescent yellow to orange.

    C. It is the fluid portion of unclotted blood.

    D. It contains only leukocytes.

22. Which statement describes serum?
    A. It results when cellular components form a fibrin clot.
    B. It is normally bright or fluorescent yellow to orange.
    C. It contains anticoagulant.
    D. It contains only leukocytes.

23. What happens to blood cells when a specimen is centrifuged?
    A. The cells lyse.
    B. The cells sink to the bottom of the tube.
    C. The cells and fluid are thoroughly mixed.
    D. Nothing happens to the specimen.

24. Which large artery or arteries carry blood to the body from the left side of the heart?
    A. vena cavae
    B. carotid
    C. mesenteric
    D. aorta

25. Which of the following veins transports blood returning to the right side of the heart from the body?
    A. coronary vein
    B. cephalic
    C. vena cavae
    D. aorta

26. How is the heart rate measured?
    A. counting respirations per minute
    B. measuring oxygen content
    C. estimating blood volume
    D. taking the pulse rate

27. What is the most common blood type?
    A. A
    B. B
    C. AB
    D. O

28. What happens if a patient receives the wrong blood transfusion?
    A. Nothing happens to the patient that is abnormal.
    B. Transfusion reactions can lead to death.
    C. White cells begin to multiply abnormally.
    D. Nerve cells contract and cause pain.

29. A "differential count" refers to:
    A. blood pressure
    B. contraction of the heart
    C. enumeration of specific types of WBCs
    D. a heart murmur

30. Which arteries supply blood to the head and neck regions?
    A. hepatic
    B. subclavian
    C. brachial
    D. carotid

31. Which of the following is the major artery in the antecubital area of the arm?
    A. brachial
    B. carotid
    C. radial
    D. aorta

32. Which of the following veins is most commonly used for venipuncture?
    A. median cubital
    B. femoral
    C. great saphenous
    D. jugular

33. The term "buffy coat" refers to:
    A. erythrocytes and platelets
    B. leukocytes and platelets
    C. mononuclear cells
    D. protein and mineral deposits

34. A phlebotomist enters a room and the patient states that she is being treated with coumadin. What does this mean for the phlebotomist?
    A. the patient may bleed excessively
    B. the patient is pregnant
    C. the blood cell count is abnormally high
    D. the phlebotomist should refer the patient to their doctor

35. Which of the following best describes the term "hemostasis"?
    A. maintenance/retention of circulating blood in the vascular system
    B. vasoconstriction to prevent blood loss
    C. a steady-state condition
    D. clot retraction

36. The term "fibrinolysis" refers to:
    A. clot retraction
    B. platelet degranulation
    C. vasoconstriction
    D. dissolution of clot and regeneration of vessel

37. Tests for blood types and cross-match testing for donor blood are done in which of the following areas of the laboratory?
    A. hematology
    B. immunohematology
    C. clinical chemistry
    D. molecular pathology

38. Which of the following represents a reference range for a platelet count?
    A. $50,000/mm^3$
    B. 50,000 to $90,000/mm^3$
    C. 95,000 to $100,000/mm^3$
    D. 200,000 to $450,000/mm^3$

39. Which of the following statements best characterizes hemophilia?
    A. fear of needles
    B. fear of the sight of blood
    C. disease caused by internal blood clots
    D. excessive bleeding owing to inadequate clotting factors

40. The longest vein in the body is the:
    A. greater saphenous
    B. median cubital
    C. aorta
    D. superior vena cava

41. How are bone marrow samples taken?
    A. aortic puncture
    B. aspiration from the iliac crest of the hip
    C. heel puncture
    D. subclavian puncture

42. A reference range for RBCs would most likely be:
    A. 4.5 to 5.5 million/mm^3
    B. 10 to 20 million/mm^3
    C. 5,000 to $9,000/mm^3$
    D. $1,000/mm^3$

43. Platelet functions are assessed in the laboratory using:
    A. anticoagulated venous blood
    B. coagulated venous blood
    C. bone marrow aspirates
    D. only capillary blood from a finger puncture

44. Hemoglobin content is assessed in the laboratory by analyzing:
    A. white blood cells
    B. erythrocytes
    C. megakaryocytes
    D. platelets

For Questions 45–50, refer to Figure 4.1.

45. The vein labeled #1 most closely resembles which of the following veins?
    A. subclavian
    B. axillary
    C. cephalic
    D. basilic

46. The vein labeled #2 most closely resembles which of the following veins?
    A. subclavian
    B. axillary
    C. cephalic
    D. brachial

47. The vein labeled #3 most closely resembles which of the following veins?
    A. subclavian
    B. axillary
    C. cephalic
    D. basilic

48. The vein labeled #4 most closely resembles which of the following veins?
    A. subclavian
    B. axillary
    C. cephalic
    D. basilic

FIGURE 4.1.

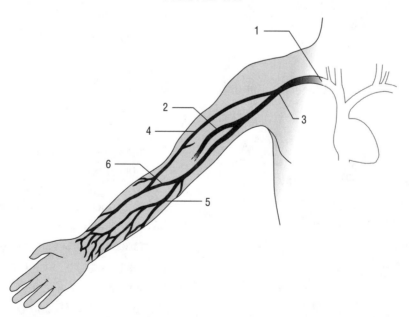

49. The vein labeled #5 most closely resembles which of the following veins?

    A. subclavian
    B. axillary
    C. cephalic
    D. basilic

50. The vein labeled #6 most closely resembles which of the following veins?

    A. median cubital
    B. axillary
    C. cephalic
    D. basilic

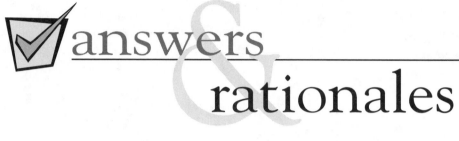

answers & rationales

1.

A. The cardiovascular system, through the circulating blood, functions to provide transportation of nutrients, gases, chemical substances, and waste removal for each cell in the body. These functions are essential for homeostasis and life maintenance. The cardiovascular system does not transport nerve impulses. (p. 92)

B, C, D. Same as above

2.

A. Capillary dialation is not an appropriate term in this context.

B. The term "systole" refers to heart contraction. (p. 92)

C. The term diastole" refers to heart relaxation.

D. The phrase "pulmonary gas exchange" refers to the transfer of oxygen and carbon dioxide in the lungs. It does not refer to heart contraction or relaxation.

3.

A. Capillary dialation is not an appropriate term in this context.

B. The term "systole" refers to heart contraction.

C. The term "diastole" refers to heart relaxation. (p. 92)

D. The phrase "pulmonary gas exchange" refers to the transfer of oxygen and carbon dioxide in the lungs. It does not refer to heart contraction or relaxation.

4.

A. Oxygen and carbon dioxide gas exchange take place in the alveoli of the lungs. (p. 95)

B. Gas exchange does not take place in the heart.

C. Gas exchange does not take place in the arteries.

D. Gas exchange does not take place in the veins.

5.

A, B, C. The average normal adult heart beats 60–80 times each minute.

D. The average normal adult heart beats 60–80 times each minute. (p. 96)

6.

A. Erythrocytes are red blood cells

B. Leukocytes are white blood cells. White blood cells are divided further into cell lines that differ in color, size, shape, and nuclear formation. Leukocytes function primarily as part of the body's defense mechanism. (p. 100)

C. Thrombocytes are platelets.

D. Sera is the plural of serum, the fluid portion of coagulated blood. The other component of coagulated blood is composed of blood cells and coagulation factors that form the fibrin clot.

7.

A. Erythrocytes are red blood cells, or RBCs. Approximately 99% of the circulating cells in the bloodstream are erythrocytes. They are biconcave disks that measure about 7 μm in diameter. Within each mature RBC are millions of hemoglobin molecules that function to carry oxygen to all parts of the body. (p. 97)

B. Leukocytes are white blood cells.

C. Thrombocytes are platelets.

D. Sera is the plural of serum, the fluid portion of coagulated blood. The other component of coagulated blood is composed of blood cells and coagulation factors that form the fibrin clot.

8.

A. Erythrocytes are red blood cells.

B. Leukocytes are white blood cells.

C. Thrombocytes are platelets. Platelets are much smaller than the other circulating cells in the bloodstream. Normally there are 250,000–450,000 platelets/mm³. Platelets help in the clotting process by transporting needed chemicals to initiate the clotting process, slowing blood loss, and assisting in the formation of a clot. (p. 101)

D. Sera is the plural of serum, the fluid portion of coagulated blood. The other component of coagulated blood is composed of blood cells and coagulation factors that form the fibrin clot.

9.

A. In a normal blood specimen from a venipuncture, venous blood is not considered highly oxygenated.

B. If a blood specimen contains an anticoagulant, then a fibrin clot will *not* form and the specimen will be plasma, which contains fibrinogen.

C. Serum is the liquid portion of the blood that remains after a blood specimen has been allowed to clot and then centrifuged. Blood cells remain meshed in a fibrin clot. It does not contain anticoagulant. (pp. 103–104)

D. Carbon monoxide is a poisonous gas.

10.

A. In a normal blood specimen from a venipuncture, venous blood is not considered highly oxygenated.

B. Plasma refers to a blood specimen that contains fibrinogen. Anticoagulants are chemical substances that prevent blood from clotting. A blood sample that has been anticoagulated can be separated by centrifugation into plasma and blood cells. (pp. 103–104)

C. If a blood specimen does not contain an anticoagulant, then a fibrin clot will form, and the specimen will be serum plus the blood clot.

D. Carbon monoxide is a poisonous gas.

11.

A. Veins carry deoxygenated blood toward the heart.

B. Arteries carry oxygenated blood away from the heart.

C. Capillaries are microscopic vessels that link arterioles to venules. They may be so small in diameter as to allow only one blood cell to pass through at any given time. Gas exchange occurs in the capillaries of tissues. (pp. 107, 110)

D. None of the blood vessels in the human body carry only white blood cells. All carry white blood cells, red blood cells, and platelets as well as other substances and chemicals necessary for sustaining life.

12.

A. Veins carry blood toward the heart (afferent vessels).

B. Arteries are vessels that carry highly oxygenated blood away from the heart (efferent vessels). They branch into smaller vessels called arterioles and into capillaries. They are normally bright red in color, have thicker elastic walls than veins do, and have a pulse. (pp. 104–109)

C. Capillaries are microscopic vessels that link arterioles and venules.

D. None of the blood vessels in the human body carry only red blood cells. All carry white blood cells, red blood cells, and platelets as well as other substances and chemicals necessary for sustaining life.

13.

A. Veins carry blood toward the heart (afferent vessels). Because the blood in veins flows against gravity in many areas of the body, these vessels have one-way valves and rely on muscular action to move blood cells through the vessels. The valves also prevent back flow of blood. All veins except the pulmonary veins contain deoxygenated blood, are dark red in color, and have thinner walls than arteries. The forearm veins that are most commonly used for venipuncture are the median cubital, basilic, and cephalic veins. (pp. 104–109)

B. Arteries carry oxygenated blood away from the heart.

C. Capillaries are microscopic vessels that link arterioles and venules.

D. None of the blood vessels in the human body carry only red blood cells. All carry white blood cells, red blood cells, and platelets as well as other substances and chemicals necessary for sustaining life.

14.

A. Erythrocytes function primarily to transport oxygen to all parts of the body.

B. The term "host cell" does not apply to any blood cells.

C. Platelets function primarily as part of the blood-clotting process.

D. Leukocytes function primarily as part of the body's defense mechanism. The cells phagocytize or ingest pathogenic microorganisms and play a role in immunity through antibody production. (p. 100)

15.

A. Erythrocytes function primarily to transport oxygen from the lungs to the tissues and carbon dioxide from the tissues to the lungs. (pp. 97–98)

B. The term "host cell" does not apply to any blood cells.

C. Platelets function primarily as part of the blood-clotting process.

D. Leukocytes, not erythrocytes, function primarily as a defense mechanism for the body.

16.

A. Erythrocytes function primarily to transport oxygen and carbon dioxide.

B. The term "host cell" does not apply to any blood cells.

C. Platelets function in the clotting process by transporting needed chemicals for clotting, forming a temporary patch or plug to slow blood loss, and contracting after the blood clot has formed. (p. 101)

D. Leukocytes function primarily as a defense mechanism for the body.

17.

A. Blood cells develop from undifferentiated stem cells in the hematopoietic or blood forming tissues such as the bone marrow. Stem cells are considered immature because they have not developed into their functional state. The cells will undergo changes in their nucleus and cytoplasm so that they differentiate and become functional once they are in the circulating blood. (p. 97)

B. The life span of each cell line differs: RBCs last about 120 days, WBCs last 1 day to several years, and platelets last 9–12 days.

C. Blood cell development does not occur in the lungs.

D. Hematopoiesis in a normal human body does not require large volumes of water.

18.

A. Red blood cells or erythrocytes measure about 7 microns in diameter, have no nuclei when circulating in the peripheral blood, and have a life span of about 120 days.

B. Red blood cells or erythrocytes measure about 7 microns in diameter, have no nuclei when circulating in the peripheral blood, and have a life span of about 120 days.

C. Red blood cells or erythrocytes measure about 7 microns in diameter, have no nuclei when circulating in the peripheral blood, and have a life span of about 120 days.

D. Red blood cells or erythrocytes are not smaller or more compact than platelets. (p. 97)

19.

A. Upper chambers of the heart are the right and left atria. (pp. 93–94)

B. The right and left ventricles are the lower chambers of the heart.

C. The inferior and superior vena cavae are the largest veins in the body. The superior vena cava brings blood from the head, neck, arms, and chest; the inferior vena cava carries deoxygenated blood from the rest of the trunk and the legs.

D. Reticulocytes are not chambers of the heart.

20.

A. There are four chambers in the human heart, which is located slightly left of the midline in the thoracic cavity. The upper chambers, or atria, are separated by the interatrial septum, and the interventricular septum divides the two ventricles, or lower chambers of the heart. (pp. 93–94)

B. There are four chambers in the human heart, which is located slightly left of the midline in the thoracic cavity. The upper chambers, or atria, are separated by the interatrial septum, and the interventricular septum divides the two ventricles, or lower chambers of the heart.

C. There are four chambers in the human heart, which is located slightly left of the midline in the thoracic cavity. The upper chambers, or atria, are separated by the interatrial septum, and the interventricular septum divides the two ventricles, or lower chambers of the heart.

D. The four chambers in the human heart are *not* called superior and inferior chambers.

21.

A. Plasma is from anticoagulated blood. It has not been allowed to form a clot.

B. Plasma is not bright yellow or fluorescent or orange.

C. The liquid portion of anticoagulated, or unclotted, blood is called plasma. It is composed of 90% water and 10% solutes, which include nutrients, amino acids, fats, metabolic wastes, respiratory gases, regulatory substances, fibrinogen, and protective substances. (p. 103)

D. Plasma does not contain "only leukocytes."

22.

A. Serum does not contain anticoagulant. Serum is the fluid portion of a blood specimen that results when cellular components form a fibrin clot. (p. 103)

B. Serum is not normally bright or fluorescent yellow or orange.

C. Serum does not contain anticoagulant.

D. Serum does not contain "only leukocytes."

23.

A. The cells do not lyse after standard specimen centrifugation.

B. The cells sink to the bottom of the tube after centrifugation because they are heavier than the liquid portion. (p. 103)

C. The cells and fluid portion are separated, not "thoroughly mixed" after centrifugation.

D. The answer "nothing happens to the specimen" is incorrect as stated above.

24.

A. The vena cavae are large veins, not arteries.

B. Right and left carotid arteries feed the head and neck regions.

C. The mesenteric artery extends into the abdominal area.

D. The aorta is the large artery that carries blood to the body from the left side of the heart. (p. 105)

25.

A. The coronary veins returns deoxygenated blood from the heart.

B. The cephalic vein returns deoxygenated blood from the arm.

C. The inferior and superior vena cavae are large veins that transport blood returning to

the right side of the heart from the body. (pp. 92–95, 106)

D. The aorta is the large artery that carries blood to the body from the left side of the heart.

26.

A. Heart rate is not measured by counting respirations.

B. Heart rate is not measured by oxygen content.

C. Heart rate is not measured by estimating blood volume.

D. Heart rate is measured by taking the pulse rate. (p. 96)

27.

A. The most common blood type is not A.

B. The most common blood type is not B.

C. The most common blood type is not AB.

D. The most common blood type is O. (p. 99)

28.

A. If a patient receives the wrong blood transfusion, many unfavorable events can occur. The answer that "nothing happens" is incorrect.

B. Transfusion reactions can occur if the wrong blood is transfused into a patient. The cells of the donor may react with antibodies of the patient, causing hemolysis, agglutination, and clogging of small blood vessels, damage to kidneys, liver, lungs, heart, or the brain. These reactions can lead to death. (p. 100)

C. White cells will not begin to multiply abnormally in this case.

D. It would not be likely that nerve cells would begin to contract and cause pain in this case.

29.

A. "Blood pressure" is not the same type of measurement as a differential count.

B. "Heart contractions" are not a differential count.

C. A differential count refers to the enumeration of specific types of WBCs. (p. 100)

D. "A heart murmur" is not a differential count.

30.

A. The hepatic artery supplies blood to the liver.

B. The subclavian arteries supply blood to the arms.

C. The brachial arteries supply blood to the arms.

D. The carotid arteries supply blood to the head region. (p. 105)

31.

A. The brachial artery is the major artery in the antecubital area of the arm. (p. 105)

B. The carotid artery transports blood to the head region.

C. The radial artery is in the lower arm.

D. The aorta is the largest artery and takes blood from the heart to the trunk of the body.

32.

A. The median cubital vein is the best for venipuncture because it is generally the largest and best-anchored vein. (p. 109)

B. The femoral vein is in the leg region and is not recommended for routine venipuncture.

C. The great saphenous vein is in the leg, and is the longest vein in the body. It is not recommended for routine venipuncture.

D. The jugular vein is in the neck region and is not recommended for venipuncture.

33.

A. Erythrocytes settle below the buffy coat and platelets are part of the buffy coat.

B. The term "buffy coat" refers to the layer of white blood cells and platelets that form when plasma is centrifuged or if the cells are allowed to settle. It forms above the red blood cells and below the plasma. (p. 103)

C. Mononuclear cells are only one type of cell within the buffy coat.

D. Protein and minerals are not found in the buffy coat.

34.

A. If the patient is on coumadin, or other anti-coagulant therapy, the phlebotomist should be on the alert that the patient might bleed more than usual. (p. 103)

B. Coumadin does not relate to pregnancy.

C. Coumadin does not cause the blood cell count to be abnormally high.

D. The phlebotomist does not have to refer the patient to the doctor in this case.

35.

A. Hemostasis is the maintenance of circulating blood in the liquid state and retention of blood in the vascular system by preventing blood loss. (p. 110)

B. Vasoconstriction to prevent blood loss is the first phase in the vascular process of minimizing blood loss. It is only one component of the hemostatic process.

C. A steady-state condition is known as homostasis.

D. Clot retraction occurs when bleeding has stopped. It is the fourth phase in the hemostatic process.

36.

A. Clot retraction is phase four of the hemostatic process.

B. Platelet degranulation occurs during the second phase of the hemostatic process.

C. Vasoconstriction is the first phase in the vascular hemostatic process.

D. In the final phase of hemostasis, fibrinolysis occurs, whereby repair and regeneration of the injured vessel take place, and the clot slowly begins to dissolve as other cells carry out further repair. (p. 111)

37.

A. The hematology laboratory performs tests related to blood cells and coagulation indices.

B. Laboratory tests for blood typing and cross-matching for donor blood are performed in the immunohematology laboratory. (p. 115)

C. The clinical chemistry laboratory performs tests related to detection of chemical substances in the serum.

D. The molecular pathology laboratory performs a variety of tests on tissues or cells using tests that detect molecular abnormalities or utilize molecular probes.

38.

A. The reference range for platelets is 250,000 to 450,000/mm^3.

B. The reference range for platelets is 250,000 to 450,000/mm^3.

C. The reference range for platelets is 250,000 to 450,000/mm^3.

D. The reference range for platelets is 250,000 to 450,000/mm^3. (p. 97)

39.

A. Fear of needles is not hemophilia; however, it is a common anxiety-producing feeling among patients before venipuncture.

B. Fear of the sight of blood is not hemophilia; however, it is a common anxiety-producing feeling among patients undergoing phlebotomy. Some individuals will faint at the sight of blood.

C. Overactive clotting can cause clots within the body, such as an embolus or thrombus.

D. Hemophilia is a disease that can cause excessive bleeding owing to abnormalities or suppressed clotting factors. (p. 115)

40.

A. The greater saphenous vein is the longest in the body. It extends the length of the leg. (p. 106)

B. The median cubital vein is a vein of the arm.

C. The aorta is a large artery extending from the heart; it is not a vein.

D. The superior vena cava is a vein connecting to the heart. It brings blood from the head, neck, arms, and chest.

41.

A. Bone marrow cannot be aspirated from the aorta.

B. Bone marrow is aspirated from the iliac crest of the hip. A physician performs the aspiration. Marrow specimens can be stained and studied microscopically for the detection of abnormal numbers and morphological characteristics of blood cells. (p. 113)

C. Bone marrow cannot be aspirated from a heel puncture.

D. Bone marrow cannot be removed from the subclavian vein.

42.

A. A reference range (sometimes referred to as the normal range) for a red blood cell count is 4.5 to 5.5 million/mm³. (p. 97)

B. Ten to 20 million cells/mm³ would be excessively high for a red cell count.

C. A count of 5,000 to 9,000 cells/mm³ is too low for a normal red cell count.

D. A count of 1,000/mm³ is too low for a normal red cell count.

43.

A. Platelet function as well as each coagulation factor can be measured from anticoagulated blood specimens in the coagulation section of the clinical hematology laboratory. (p. 113)

B. Coagulated venous blood cannot be used to assess platelet function, since the clotting sequence utilizes the platelets.

C. Bone marrow aspirates cannot be used to assess platelet functions that occur in the peripheral blood. Platelets in the bone marrow are not fully mature and would function very differently.

D. Platelet functions and/or coagulation tests can be performed on finger puncture blood but it is not the only source of a specimen.

44.

A. White blood cells cannot be used to determine hemoglobin concentration because they do not contain hemoglobin.

B. Since hemoglobin is contained within the red blood cells, they must be lysed to release the hemoglobin for assessment. (p. 113)

C. Megakaryocytes cannot be used to determine hemoglobin concentration because they do not contain hemoglobin.

D. Platelets cannot be used to determine hemoglobin concentration because they do not contain hemoglobin.

FIGURE 4.1. Major arm veins.

1. **Subclavian vein**
2. **Brachial vein**
3. **Axillary vein**
4. **Cephalic vein**
5. **Basilic vein**
6. **Median cubital vein**

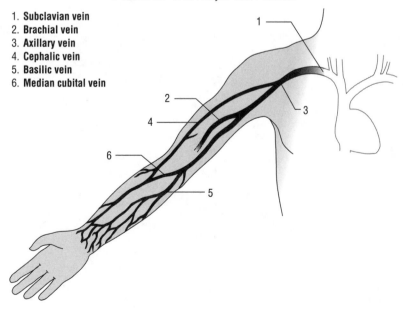

For Questions 45–50, refer to Figure 4.1.

45.

A. The vein labeled #1 most closely resembles the subclavian vein. (p. 110)

46.

D. The vein labeled #2 most closely resembles the brachial vein. (p. 110)

47.

B. The vein labeled #3 most closely resembles the axillary vein. (p. 110)

48.

C. The vein labeled #4 most closely resembles the cephalic vein. (p. 110)

49.

D. The vein labeled #5 most closely resembles the basilic vein. (p. 110)

50.

A. The vein labeled #6 most closely resembles the median cubital vein. (p. 110)

5 Infection Control

chapter objectives

Upon completion of Chapter 5, the learner is responsible for the following:

➤ Define the term health care-acquired (nosocomial) infection.

➤ Identify the basic programs for infection control.

➤ Explain the proper techniques for hand-washing, gowning, gloving, masking, double bagging, and entering and exiting the various isolation areas.

➤ Identify the potential routes of infection and methods for preventing transmission of microorganisms through these routes.

➤ Identify steps to avoid transmission of bloodborne pathogens.

➤ Describe the various isolation procedures and reasons for their use.

DIRECTIONS Each of the questions or incomplete statements below is followed by four suggested answers or completions. Select one answer that is best in each case.

1. What percent of all hospitalized patients in the United States acquire nosocomial (health care-acquired) infections?
   A. 1%
   B. 5%
   C. 10%
   D. 20%

2. Which of the following is *not* a component that makes up the chain of infection?
   A. mode of transmission
   B. susceptible host
   C. mode of transportation
   D. source

3. Which of the following is considered a fomite?
   A. transfusions
   B. hand-washing
   C. immunizations
   D. scrub suits

4. Good nutrition can break the chain of nosocomial infections between the:
   A. source and mode of transmission
   B. mode of transportation and susceptible host
   C. source and susceptible host
   D. mode of transmission and susceptible host

5. In Spanish, *peligro biologico* refers to the English term:
   A. hepatitis
   B. bloodborne pathogen

C. *Salmonella*
D. biohazardous

6. Which type of isolation precaution is frequently required for patients with infections that are transmitted through colonized microorganisms by direct hand contact?
   A. droplet precautions
   B. skin isolation
   C. reverse isolation
   D. contact precautions

7. Which of the following diseases usually require(s) airborne precautions?
   A. herpes simplex
   B. wound infections
   C. pertussis
   D. tuberculosis

8. Which of the following interrupts the link between the susceptible host to the chain of infection?
   A. gene splicing
   B. radiation therapy
   C. chemotherapy
   D. good nutrition

9. The work status of a health care provider should be "off from work" if he or she has:
   A. chicken pox
   B. herpes simplex
   C. hepatitis C
   D. gonorrhea

10. Which of the following illnesses is usually transmitted from one person to another by coughing or sneezing?

    A. scabies

    B. weeping dermatitis

    C. diphtheria

    D. impetigo caused by *Staphylococcus*

11. Vectors in transmitting infectious diseases include:

    A. rabies

    B. *Salmonella*

    C. mites

    D. age

12. Babies whose mothers have which of the following problems must be isolated from other infants?

    A. genital herpes

    B. kidney failure and are in a dialysis unit

    C. burns

    D. cancer

13. A "health care-acquired" infection occurs when:

    A. the chain of infection is complete

    B. a source is detected

    C. a means of transmission is maintained by disinfectants

    D. a susceptible host remains stable

14. Disinfectants are:

    A. quaternary ammonium compounds

    B. chemicals that are used to inhibit the growth and development of microorganisms but do not necessarily kill them

    C. chemicals that are used to remove or kill pathogenic microorganisms

    D. used frequently on skin

15. Which of the following is a commonly occurring pathogenic agent that causes health care-acquired (nosocomial) infections of the gastrointestinal tract?

    A. *Haemophilus vaginalis*

    B. *Vibrio cholerae*

    C. *Neisseria gonorrhoeae*

    D. *Bordetella pertussis*

16. Which of the following microorganisms normally found in the GI tract causes health care-acquired bladder infections?

    A. malaria

    B. tuberculosis

    C. *Escherichia coli*

    D. smallpox

17. Which of the following chemical compounds is an antiseptic for skin?

    A. Hexylresorcinol

    B. ethylene oxide

    C. 1% phenol

    D. chlorophenol

18. A commonly identified causative agent of health care-acquired infections in the nursery unit is:

    A. *Escherichia coli*

    B. *Shigella*

    C. *Vibrio cholerae*

    D. *Haemophilus vaginalis*

19. Reverse isolation is commonly used for patients who have:

    A. *Vibrio cholerae*

    B. hepatitis A

    C. immunodeficiency disorders

    D. whooping cough

20. Which of the following is a commonly identified pathogenic microorganism that causes health care-acquired skin infections?
    A. *Candida albicans*
    B. *Haemophilus vaginalis*
    C. *Haemophilus influenzae*
    D. *Moraxella lacunata*

21. Antiseptics for skin include:
    A. hypochlorite solution
    B. formaldehyde
    C. ethylene oxide
    D. iodine

22. Which of the following chemicals has the fastest speed of action in hand-hygiene antiseptic cleaning?
    A. iodophors
    B. phenol derivatives
    C. chlorhexidine
    D. 70% isopropyl alcohol

23. Which of the following types of health care-acquired (nosocomial) infections can be caused by any microorganism in sufficient numbers?
    A. dermal infections
    B. wound infections
    C. urinary tract infections
    D. respiratory infections

24. Under the CDC isolation guidelines, three sets of precautions include:
    A. airborne, droplet, and contact
    B. enteric, contact, and respiratory
    C. airborne, respiratory, and contact
    D. complete, droplet, and airborne

25. Using the CDC isolation guidelines, bloodborne pathogen precautions have been grouped into:

    A. contact isolation technique, complete isolation technique, and tuberculosis isolation
    B. complete isolation technique and body substance isolation
    C. universal precautions and body substance isolation
    D. standard precautions and expanded precautions

26. Which of the following isolation techniques requires that any blood collection equipment taken into the patient's room must be taken out after the blood is collected?
    A. droplet precautions
    B. reverse isolation
    C. contact precautions
    D. A and C

27. The following hand-hygiene antiseptic agent is most effective for *Mycobacterium tuberculosis:*
    A. iodophors
    B. isopropyl alcohol
    C. phenol
    D. quaternary ammonium

28. A factor that increases a host's susceptibility in the chain of infection is:
    A. use of disposable equipment
    B. proper nutrition
    C. an immunization
    D. drug use

29. Contact precautions may be required for patients infected with:
    A. infectious tuberculosis
    B. herpes simplex
    C. rubella
    D. measles

30. A phlebotomist had to avoid contact with patients for 24 hours after being started on an appropriate antibiotic and appearing symptom-free. What type of infection could he or she have acquired for the above work limitations to apply?
    A. measles
    B. rubella
    C. chicken pox
    D. strep throat (group A)

31. In health care facilities, which is a typical fomite?
    A. 70% isopropyl alcohol
    B. hexachlorophene
    C. phlebotomy tray
    D. iodine for blood culture collections

32. In the process of preparing to enter a patient's room in isolation, which of the following would occur first?
    A. donning gloves and positioning them
    B. donning mask
    C. discarding mask
    D. untying gown at the neck

33. Which of the following is the most important procedure in the prevention of disease transmission in health care institutions?
    A. reporting personal illnesses to supervisor
    B. hand-washing
    C. use of personal protection equipment
    D. use of appropriate waste disposal practices

34. Which of the following would require droplet precautions?
    A. *Mycoplasma pneumonia*
    B. *Shigella*
    C. *E. coli*
    D. *Clostridium difficile*

35. Which of the following is designed to reduce the risk of transmission of microorganisms from both recognized and unrecognized sources of infection in health care facilities?
    A. standard precautions
    B. enteric isolation
    C. complete isolation
    D. drainage/secretion isolation

36. Which of the following organizations requires the development and implementation of an infection control program in a health care facility?
    A. ASCP
    B. CLT
    C. CLIA
    D. JCAHO

37. Health care-acquired infections occur when what is complete?
    A. infection control surveillance
    B. an employee health monitoring program
    C. chain of infection
    D. a nosocomial infection

38. What, as part of the U.S. Public Health Service, oversees the investigation of various diseases?
    A. CLSI
    B. FDA
    C. CDC
    D. JCAHO

39. What infectious agent affecting a patient requires the use of a personal respirator by the phlebotomist?
    A. *Escherichia coli*
    B. *Mycobacterium tuberculosis*
    C. *Shigella*
    D. *Salmonella*

40. Which of the following laboratory-acquired infections is most prevalent?
    A. Rocky Mountain spotted fever
    B. amebic dysentery
    C. HIV infection
    D. *E. coli*

41. If an accident occurs, such as a needlestick, the injured health care provider should immediately:
    A. contact his or her immediate supervisor
    B. fill out the necessary health care forms
    C. take the needle back to the clinical laboratory for verification of the accident
    D. cleanse the area with isopropyl alcohol and apply an adhesive bandage

42. To prevent skin and mucous membrane exposure when contact with a patient's blood is anticipated, the following should be worn.
    A. BBP
    B. PPE
    C. CDC
    D. FDA

43. Health care-acquired infections are also referred to as:
    A. nonpathogenic
    B. bloodborne pathogens
    C. nosocomial infections
    D. aseptic

44. When collecting blood from neonates in the nursery, what health care-acquired infection is highly prevalent in this area?
    A. Rotavirus
    B. Smallpox
    C. Measles
    D. *Vibrio cholerae*

45. An outbreak of particular health care-acquired infections in a health care facility is detected through:
    A. the clinical chemistry department
    B. infection control surveillance
    C. personnel records
    D. individuals transmitting fomites

46. Therapeutic measures (i.e., chemotherapy, radiation therapy) in a patient create what part of the chain of infection?
    A. pathogen
    B. source
    C. mode of transmission
    D. susceptible host

47. Proper hand-washing prior to and after blood collection requires rubbing wet, soapy hands together vigorously for at least:
    A. 5 seconds
    B. 15 seconds
    C. 1 minute
    D. 2 minutes

48. In addition to standard precautions, use contact precautions for patients with known:
    A. *Haemophilus influenzae*
    B. wound infections
    C. rubella
    D. mumps

49. Which of the following requires respiratory protective equipment for the phlebotomist?
    A. standard precautions
    B. droplet precautions
    C. airborne precautions
    D. contact precautions

50. After completion of blood collection in an isolation room, which of the following steps should occur last?

    A. the gloves are removed
    B. the mask is removed
    C. wash hands
    D. the gown is removed

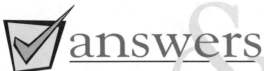

answers & rationales

1.

A, C, D. These percentages (1%, 10%, 20%) are incorrect.

B. Five percent of all hospitalized patients in the United States acquire health care-acquired infections. (p. 124)

2.

A. The three components that make up the chain are the source, mode of transmission, and susceptible host.

B. The three components that make up the chain are the source, mode of transmission, and susceptible host.

C. The three components that make up the chain are the source, mode of transmission, and susceptible host. (p. 130)

D. The three components that make up the chain are the source, mode of transmission, and susceptible host.

3.

A. Transfusions are given to interrupt the chain of nosocomial infections and are not fomites. Scrub suits, computer keyboards, doorknobs, and telephones are a few examples of fomites.

B. Hand-washing is performed to interrupt the infectious process of nosocomial infections and therefore is not a fomite. Scrub suits, computer keyboards, doorknobs, and telephones are a few examples of fomites.

C. Immunizations interrupt the infection process. Scrub suits, computer keyboards, doorknobs, and telephones are a few examples of fomites.

D. Scrub suits, computer keyboards, doorknobs, and telephones are a few examples of fomites (objects that can harbor infectious agents and transmit infections). (p. 131)

4.

A. Good nutrition is an important factor in interrupting the chain of nosocomial infections between the source and susceptible host.

B. Good nutrition is an important factor in interrupting the chain of nosocomial infections between the source and susceptible host.

C. Good nutrition is an important factor in interrupting the chain of nosocomial infections between the source and susceptible host. (pp. 130–132)

D. Good nutrition is an important factor in interrupting the chain of nosocomial infections between the source and susceptible host.

5.

A, B, C. In Spanish, *peligro biologico* refers to the English term "biohazardous," not hepatitis, bloodborne pathogen, or *Salmonella*.

D. In Spanish, *peligro biologico* refers to the English term "biohazardous." (Joyce, 2000)

6.

A. Droplet precautions prevent transmission of large-particle droplets in the air such as in coughing from diphtheria.

B. Skin isolation is not a type of isolation.

C. Patients are put in reverse isolation not because they have an infection, but because they are highly susceptible to infection and need to be protected from the external environment.

D. Contact precautions prevent transmission of known or suspected infected or colonized microorganisms by direct hand or skin to skin contact for conditions such as in hepatitis A. (p. 138)

7.

A. A person with a herpes simplex infection would be placed in contact precautions.

B. A person with wound infections would be placed in contact precautions.

C. A person with a pertussis infection would be placed in droplet precautions.

D. A person with a tuberculosis infection would have airborne precautions to reduce the spread of airborne droplet transmission. (p. 138)

8.

A. Gene splicing is a new treatment involving DNA resynthesis in the patient. However, it is not used to interrupt the chain of nosocomial infection.

B. Radiation therapy is a treatment to destroy cancerous growths in patients but is not considered a factor in the chain of nosocomial infection.

C. Chemotherapy is an agent that interrupts growth of cancerous cells but is not considered a factor in the chain of nosocomial infection.

D. Good nutrition interrupts the chain of nosocomial infection between the susceptible host and the source. (pp. 129–132)

9.

A. For 7 days after eruption of chicken pox, the employee should not work. (p. 129)

B. An employee who has herpes simplex may work.

C. An employee who has hepatitis C may work as long as his or her blood or body fluids are not exposed to anyone else.

D. An employee having gonorrhea may work.

10.

A. Scabies is a skin infection caused by mites, not by microscopic airborne droplets.

B. Weeping dermatitis is a skin disorder usually caused by an allergic response (i.e., wearing gloves).

C. Diphtheria infection leads to droplet precautions due to coughing. (p. 134)

D. Impetigo is a systemic infection caused by *Staphylococcus* and is transmitted through direct contact, not airborn droplets.

11.

A. Rabies is a disease caused by a virus, whereas a vector is an insect or rodent that carries and transmits infectious diseases.

B. *Salmonella* is a type of bacteria, not a vector.

C. Mites act as vectors in transmitting infectious diseases. (p. 130)

D. Age is not a vector. Vectors are insects and rodents that carry and transmit infectious diseases.

12.

A. Babies whose mothers have genital herpes must be isolated from other infants. (p. 142)

B. Babies whose mothers have genital herpes must be isolated from other infants.

C. A baby whose mother has been burned is not isolated, but the mother may have to be isolated to protect her from obtaining an infection.

D. Babies whose mothers have genital herpes must be isolated from other infants.

13.

A. Health care-acquired infections occur when the chain of infection is complete. The three components that make up the chain are the source, mode of transmission, and susceptible host. (p. 132)

B. Health care-acquired infections occur when the chain of infection is complete. The three components that make up the chain are source, mode of transmission, and susceptible host.

C. Health care-acquired infections occur when the chain of infection is complete. The three components that make up the chain are source, mode of transmission, and susceptible host.

D. Health care-acquired infections occur when the chain of infection is complete. The three components that make up the chain are source, mode of transmission, and susceptible host.

14.

A. Quaternary ammonium compounds are antiseptics for skin that are found in many soaps.

B. Antiseptics are chemicals that are used to inhibit the growth and development of microorganisms but do not necessarily kill them.

C. Disinfectants are chemical compounds that are used to remove or kill pathogenic microorganisms (p. 151)

D. Disinfectants are strong chemicals and are not used frequently on skin.

15.

A. *Haemophilus vaginalis* is a microorganism that causes health care-acquired infections in the genital tract.

B. *Vibrio cholerae* is a pathogenic agent that causes health care-acquired infections of the gastrointestinal tract. (p. 126)

C. *Neisseria gonorrhoeae* is a pathogenic agent that causes health care-acquired infections in the eye.

D. *Bordetella pertussis* is a bacteria that causes health care-acquired infections in the respiratory tract.

16.

A. Malaria is not normally found in the GI tract.

B. Tuberculosis is caused by a *Mycobacterium* that usually affects the lungs.

C. Urinary tract health care-acquired infections are frequently caused by *Escherichia coli*. (pp. 124, 126)

D. Smallpox does not lead to health care-acquired bladder infections.

17.

A. Hexylresorcinol is an antiseptic for skin that is used frequently in surgery. (p. 152)

B. Ethylene oxide is a disinfectant and toxic for skin use.

C. 1% phenol is a disinfectant and is not used on skin.

D. Chlorophenol is a disinfectant and toxic for skin use.

18.

A. *Escherichia coli* is a commonly identified pathogenic agent that causes nosocomial infections in the nursery unit. (p. 127)

B. *Shigella* is a commonly identified pathogenic microorganism that causes nosocomial infections in the gastrointestinal tract.

C. *Vibrio cholerae* is a commonly identified pathogenic microorganism that causes nosocomial infections in the gastrointestinal tract.

D. *Haemophilus vaginalis* is a commonly identified pathogenic microorganism that causes nosocomial infections in the genital tract.

19.

A. Contact precautions are used for patients with infections that are transmitted by ingestion of the pathogen causing diarrheal diseases such as *Vibrio cholerae*.

B. Contact precautions are used for patients with infections that are transmitted by ingestion of the pathogen causing diarrheal diseases such as hepatitis A.

C. Reverse, or protective, isolation is used for patients who have immunodeficiency disorders to protect them from external environments. (p. 141)

D. Droplet precautions are required for patients with infections that may be transmitted by air droplets such as in whooping cough.

20.

A. *Candida albicans* is a commonly identified pathogenic agent that causes health care-acquired skin infections. (pp. 126–127)

B. *Haemophilus vaginalis* is a pathogenic microorganism that causes genital tract infections.

C. *Haemophilus influenzae* is a pathogenic microorganism that causes health care-acquired ear infections.

D. *Moraxella lacunata* is a commonly identified pathogenic agent that causes health care-acquired eye infections.

21.

A. Hypochlorite solutions are disinfectants used on surfaces and instruments for cleansing but not skin because of their corrosive effects to skin.

B. Formaldehyde is a disinfectant having noxious fumes.

C. Ethylene oxide is a disinfectant that is toxic and corrosive for cleansing the skin.

D. Iodine solutions are commonly used to cleanse the skin for blood culture collections. (pp. 152–153)

22.

A. Alcohols have the fastest speed of action for hand-hygiene antiseptic cleaning.

B. Alcohols have the fastest speed of action for hand-hygiene antiseptic cleaning.

C. Alcohols have the fastest speed of action for hand-hygiene antiseptic cleaning.

D. Alcohols (e.g., isopropyl alcohol) have the fastest speed of action for hand-hygiene antiseptic cleaning. (p. 141)

23.

A, B, D. Dermal, wound, or respiratory infections are usually caused by specified pathogenic organisms.

C. Urinary tract infections are the most prevalent of nosocomial infections and can be caused by any microorganism in sufficient numbers. (p. 126)

24.

A. Under the most recent CDC isolation guidelines, three sets of precautions include airborne, droplet, and contact. (p. 132)

B, C, D. Under the CDC isolation guidelines, the old categories of isolation and disease-specific precautions have been collapsed into three sets of precautions that include airborne, droplet, and contact.

25.

A, B, C. While some of these terms were used previously, the CDC isolation guidelines have now been grouped into "standard precautions" and "expanded precautions."

D. Under the CDC isolation guidelines, the bloodborne pathogen precautions have been grouped into "standard precautions" and "expanded precautions." (p. 132)

26.

A. Except for protective (reverse) isolation, any of the transmission-based precautions require that any articles contaminated with potentially infected material in the isolation room must be left there.

B. Except for protective (reverse) isolation, any of the transmission-based precautions require that any articles contaminated with potentially infected material in the isolation room must be left there.

C. Except for protective (reverse) isolation, any of the transmission-based precautions require that any articles contaminated with potentially infected material in the isolation room must be left there.

D. Except for protective (reverse) isolation, any of the transmission-based precautions require that any articles contaminated with potentially infected material in the isolation room must be left there. (pp. 132–142)

27.

A. Iodophors are most effective against bacteria.

B. Alcohols and iodine compounds are most effective for *Mycobacterium tuberculosis*. (p. 153)

C. Phenols are most effective against Gram-positive bacteria.

D. Alcohols and iodine compounds are most effective for *Mycobacterium tuberculosis*.

28.

A. Use of disposable equipment decreases the chances of infections, since the disposable equipment is sterile or chemically clean.

B. Proper nutrition increases the host's resistance to infections.

C. Immunizations increase the immune response of a person to infectious diseases and decrease the chance of infections.

D. Drug use is definitely a factor that affects a host's susceptibility to infection, since drug use decreases the status of the person's immune resistance. (p. 131)

29.

A. Tuberculosis infections placed under airborne precautions isolation is indicated for patients with infectious tuberculosis.

B. Contact precautions are used for herpes simplex. (p. 134)

C. Droplet precautions are used for rubella infections.

D. Measles infections are placed under airborne precautions.

30.

A. If a worker has measles, he or she must remain off work a minimum of 4 days or until the rash clears.

B. If a worker has rubella, he or she must not work for a minimum of 5 days or until the rash clears.

C. If a worker has chicken pox, he or she must not work for 7 days after eruption first appears, provided lesions are dry and crusted when he or she returns.

D. Strep throat (Group A) requires that the employee be placed on appropriate antibiotics for 24 hours before he or she may come to work. (p. 129)

31.

A. 70% isopropyl alcohol is an antiseptic.

B. Hexachlorophene is an antiseptic.

C. Objects that can harbor infectious agents and transmit infection are called fomites. (p. 128)

D. Iodine for blood culture collection is an antiseptic.

32.

A. After gowning, a mask (if necessary) may be put over the nose and mouth. Then, gloves should be put on and pulled over the ends of gown sleeves.

B. After gowning, a mask (if necessary) may be put over the nose and mouth. Then, gloves should be put on and pulled over the ends of gown sleeves. (pp. 146–147)

C. After gowning, a mask (if necessary) may be put over the nose and mouth. Then, gloves should be put on and pulled over the ends of gown sleeves.

D. After gowning, a mask (if necessary) may be put over the nose and mouth. Then, gloves should be put on and pulled over the ends of gown sleeves.

33.

A, C, D. Even though these factors are very helpful and important, hand washing (hand decontamination) is the most important procedure in the prevention of disease transmission in health care facilities.

B. Hand-washing is the most important procedure in the prevention of disease transmission in health care facilities. In any isolation procedures, it should be the first and last step. (pp. 124, 131, 132)

34.

A. *Mycoplasma pneumonia* requires droplet precautions. (pp. 132, 138)

B. *Shigella* infection requires contact precautions.

C. *E. coli* infection requires contact precautions.

D. *Clostridium difficile* infection requires contact precautions.

35.

A. Standard precautions are designed to reduce the risk of transmission of microorganisms from both recognized and unrecognized sources of infection in health care facilities. (p. 132)

B. Enteric isolation is required for patients with recognizable infections that are transmitted by ingestion of a pathogen.

C. Complete isolation is required for patients having a recognizable contagious disease such as rabies or chicken pox.

D. Drainage/secretion isolation is required after surgery or if a patient is admitted with a skin infection. It is required only for a recognized source of infection.

36.

A. The Joint Commission on Accreditation of Healthcare Organizations (JCAHO) requires the development and implementation of an infection control program in a health care facility.

B. The Joint Commission on Accreditation of Healthcare Organizations (JCAHO) requires the development and implementation of an infection control program in a health care facility.

C. The Joint Commission on Accreditation of Healthcare Organizations (JCAHO) requires the development and implementation of an infection control program in a health care facility.

D. The Joint Commission on Accreditation of Healthcare Organizations (JCAHO) requires the development and implementation of an infection control program in a health care facility. (p. 124)

37.

A. Health care-acquired infections occur when the chain of infection is complete.

B. Health care-acquired infections occur when the chain of infection is complete.

C. Health care-acquired infections occur when the chain of infection is complete. (p. 127)

D. Health care-acquired infections occur when the chain of infection is complete.

38.

A. The Centers for Disease Control and Prevention (CDC), as part of the U.S. Public Health Service, oversees the investigation and control of various diseases.

B. The Centers for Disease Control and Prevention (CDC), as part of the U.S. Public Health Service, oversees the investigation and control of various diseases.

C. The Centers for Disease Control and Prevention (CDC), as part of the U.S. Public Health Service, oversees the investigation and control of various diseases. (p. 124)

D. The Centers for Disease Control and Prevention (CDC), as part of the U.S. Public Health Service, oversees the investigation and control of various diseases.

39.

A, C, D. *E. coli, Shigella,* and *Salmonella* can be infectious but would not require the use of a personal respirator.

B. *Mycobacterium tuberculosis* causes a lung infection that can lead to airborne transmission to someone else. Thus, a personal respirator is required to be used by the health care worker when providing care to a patient with this infection. (p. 135)

40.

A. Laboratory personnel have a high incidence of hepatitis B, tuberculosis, tularemia, and Rocky Mountain spotted fever. (pp. 142–143)

B, C, D. Amebic dysentery, HIV infection, or *E. coli* infections are not most prevalent among laboratory personnel.

41.

A. If an accident occurs, such as a needlestick, the health care provider should immediately cleanse the area with isopropyl alcohol and apply a bandage. He or she can then contact a supervisor.

B. Filling out the necessary health forms is important, but it is *not* the most immediate action required.

C. If an accident occurs, such as a needlestick, the actual needle is *not* required for verification. In fact, it is a biohazard.

D. If an accident occurs, such as a needlestick, the health care provider should immediately cleanse the area with isopropyl alcohol and apply a bandage. (p. 128)

42.

A, C, D. BBP, CDC, and FDA are not appropriate answers.

B. Personal protective equipment (PPE) are barriers (i.e., gloves, facial masks, respirators, etc.) that should be worn to prevent skin and mucous membrane exposure when contact with a patient's blood is anticipated. (p. 135)

43.

A. Nonpathogenic refers to nondisease.

B. Bloodborne pathogens (BBPs) are used to described infectious microorganisms present in blood and other body fluids.

C. Nosocomial (health care-acquired) infections are those that are acquired by a patient after admission to a health care facility. (p. 124)

D. Aseptic is a term that means without organisms and infections.

44.

A. Rotavirus is a highly prevalent health care-acquired infection in the nursery unit of a health care facility. (p. 127)

B, C, D. Smallpox, measles, and *vibrio cholerae* are *not* highly prevalent in a neonatal nursery.

45.

A, C, D. Neither the clinical chemistry department, personnel records, nor individuals can accomplish an outbreak investigation. It requires an Infection Control surveillance program.

B. An outbreak of particular health care-acquired infections in a health care facility is detected through infection control surveillance. (p. 141)

46.

A, B, C. Therapeutic measures do not usually create the pathogen, source, or mode of transmission in the "chain of infection."

D. Therapeutic measures (i.e., chemotherapy, radiation therapy) in a patient create the "susceptible host" in the chain of infection. (p. 131)

47.

A. Proper hand-washing, prior to and after blood collection, requires rubbing wet, soapy hands together vigorously for at least 15 seconds.

B. Proper hand-washing, prior to and after blood collection, requires rubbing wet, soapy hands together vigorously for at least 15 seconds. (p. 140)

C. Proper hand-washing, prior to and after blood collection, requires rubbing wet, soapy hands together vigorously for at least 15 seconds.

D. Proper hand-washing, prior to and after blood collection, requires rubbing wet, soapy hands together vigorously for at least 15 seconds.

48.

A. Airborne precautions are used for patients infected with *Haemophilus influenzae.*

B. Contact precautions are used for patients with wound infections. (p. 134)

C. Droplet precautions are used for patients with rubella.

D. Droplet precautions are used for patients with mumps.

49.

A, B, D. Standard, droplet, and contact precautions do not require respiratory protective equipment.

C. Respiratory protective equipment for the phlebotomist is required for airborne precautions. (p. 134)

50.

A, B, D. Gloves, mask, and gown removal are *not* the last steps after blood collection in an isolation room.

C. After completion of blood collection in an isolation room, the gown is first untied, followed by the gloves being removed. Then the gown is taken off, followed by the mask, and finally the hands are washed. (pp. 148–149)

6 Safety and First Aid

chapter objectives

Upon completion of Chapter 6, the learner is responsible for the following:

➤ Discuss safety awareness for health care workers.

➤ Explain the measures that should be taken for fire, electrical, radiation, mechanical, and chemical safety in a health care facility.

➤ Describe the essential elements of a disaster emergency plan for a health care facility.

➤ Explain the safety policies and procedures that must be followed in all phases of specimen collection and transportation.

➤ Describe the safe use of equipment in health care facilities.

➤ List three precautions that can reduce the risk of injury to patients.

DIRECTIONS Each of the questions or incomplete statements below is followed by four suggested answers or completions. Select one answer that is best in each case.

1. Safe working conditions must be ensured by the employer and have been mandated by law under the:
   A. Occupational Safety and Health Administration standards
   B. Institutional Safety and Health Act
   C. Health Care Facility Institutional Safety Act
   D. Health Care Facility and Occupational Safety Act

2. The health care provider is most likely to encounter which of the following hazards upon entering the nuclear medicine department to obtain a blood specimen from a patient?
   A. a fire hazard
   B. a radiation hazard
   C. a mechanical hazard
   D. an electrical hazard

3. If a health care provider is in an area of the health care facility where a fire starts, he or she should *first:*
   A. attempt to extinguish the fire, using the proper equipment
   B. pull the lever in the fire alarm box
   C. close all the doors and windows before leaving the area
   D. block the entrances so that others will not enter the fire area

4. For safety in the health care facility, which of the following should *not* occur?
   A. Needles, syringes, and lancets should be disposed of in a special sturdy container.
   B. Gloves should not be worn if the phlebotomist is allergic to latex.
   C. The specimen collection area should be disinfected periodically according to the clinical laboratory schedule.
   D. The patients' specimens should be covered at all times during transportation.

5. Which of the following organizations regulates the disposal of waste?
   A. EPA
   B. CLSI
   C. NFPA
   D. JCAHO

6. The first step in controlling severe bleeding is to:
   A. send for medical assistance
   B. start cardiopulmonary resuscitation
   C. apply pressure directly over the wound or venipuncture site
   D. make the individual lie down and apply pressure to the person's forehead

7. If a health care provider is caught in a fire in the health care institution, he or she should *not:*
   A. run
   B. close all the doors and windows before leaving the area
   C. attempt to extinguish the fire if it is small
   D. call the assigned fire number

8. If a chemical is spilled onto a health care worker, he or she should first:
   A. rub vigorously with one hand
   B. wait to see whether it starts to burn the skin
   C. rinse the area with a neutral chemical
   D. rinse the area with water

9. Chemicals that are defined as "explosive flammables" must be stored:
   A. in a separate storage room
   B. in small carrying containers
   C. on a high shelf away from light and heat
   D. in an explosion-proof or fireproof room or cabinet

10. According to the hazard labeling system developed by NFPA, the yellow quadrant of the diamond indicates a:
    A. flammability hazard
    B. health hazard
    C. instability hazard
    D. specific hazard

11. The hazardous labeling system developed by the NFPA has the blue quadrant of the diamond to indicate a:
    A. flammability hazard
    B. health hazard
    C. instability hazard
    D. specific hazard

12. If an electrical accident occurs involving electrical shock to an employee or a patient, the *first* thing that the health care worker should do is:
    A. move the victim
    B. shut off electrical power
    C. start CPR
    D. place a blanket over the victim

13. What are the major principles of self-protection from radiation exposure?
    A. distance, combustibility, and shielding
    B. time, distance, and shielding
    C. anticorrosive, shielding, and distance
    D. combustibility, anticorrosive, and distance

14. MSDSs must be supplied to employees according to the:
    A. Hazard Communication Standard (29 CFR 1910.1200)
    B. Environmental Protection Agency
    C. NFPA
    D. CDC

15. The first step in giving mouth-to-mouth resuscitation is to:
    A. open the airway by checking for obstructions
    B. listen and feel for return of air from the victim's mouth
    C. determine whether the victim is conscious by gently shaking the victim and yelling, "Are you okay?"
    D. look for the victim's chest to rise and fall

16. For chemical safety in the health care facility:
    A. Chemicals should be stored at least above eye level for easy visibility.
    B. It is not advisable to use aprons in addition to laboratory coats for protection against chemicals.
    C. An acid carrier should be used when transporting alkalis.
    D. Only explosives that may create a fire should be stored in an explosion-proof room.

17. An action that is recommended if first aid is given to a shock victim is:
    A. Give fluids to the victim in order to keep him or her hydrated.
    B. Place cold packs around the victim to slow his or her metabolism down, which will decrease further injury.
    C. Keep the victim lying down.
    D. Elevate the victim's head so that it is higher than the trunk of the body.

18. OSHA requires adherence to what when health care workers respond to emergencies that provide exposure to blood?
    A. Federal Drug Administration (FDA)
    B. Clinical Laboratory Standards Institute
    C. NFPA
    D. standard precautions

19. If blood has been spilled, what action should occur by the phlebotomist?
    A. Call 911 or the hospital's emergency number.
    B. Use 1:10 bleach solution or commercially prepared solution to clean it up.
    C. Keep the 1:10 bleach solution in contact with the contaminated area for a minimum of 2 minutes.
    D. Do not use gloves since they will disintegrate when cleaning the spill.

20. If an accidental needle stick injury occurs to a phlebotomist, what laboratory tests must be performed on this phlebotomist at periodic intervals?
    A. CBC and hemoglobin
    B. HIV and HCV
    C. blood pH
    D. PT and PTT

21. MSDS is an abbreviation for:
    A. Material Serum Data Sheets
    B. Material Safety Drug Sheets
    C. Material Safety Data Sheets
    D. Material Serum Drug Sheets

22. What organization developed a labeling system for hazardous chemicals that is frequently used in health care facilities?
    A. FDA
    B. NFPA
    C. CDC
    D. CLSI

23. Which of the following can serve as patient identifiers for phlebotomists to check prior to blood collection?
    A. patient's name, patient's room number
    B. patient's date of birth, patient's location
    C. patient's ID number, patient's address
    D. patient's hospital room, patient's date of birth

24. Which of the following PPE can be used without precautionary evaluation when the phlebotomist must enter a latex-safe environment?
    A. gloves
    B. laboratory coat
    C. tourniquet
    D. syringe

25. For Class A fires, what type of fire extinguishers can be used?
    A. carbon dioxide, dry chemical
    B. dry chemical, pressurized water
    C. halon, dry chemical
    D. carbon dioxide, halon

26. The chemicals with a blue storage code indicates they
    A. are highly corrosive
    B. may detonate
    C. are a health hazard
    D. are flammable

27. In times of an emergency, a tourniquet should be used to control bleeding for:
    A. a cut that is bleeding on the lower arm
    B. an amputated leg
    C. a leg that has a cut to the ankle area
    D. an arm that is lacerated above the elbow.

28. A fire that occurs near electrical equipment is classified as what type of fire?
    A. Class A
    B. Class B
    C. Class C
    D. Class D

29. A solution of bleach used for cleaning the specimen collection area is at what concentration?
    A. 1:1
    B. 1:2
    C. 1:10
    D. 1:20

30. When using a fire extinguisher, the operator should try to remember the acronym:
    A. OSHA
    B. PASS
    C. JCAHO
    D. CDC

31. OSHA stands for:
    A. Occupational Standards and Health Administration
    B. Occupational Safety and Health Administration
    C. Occupational Safety and Hazards Administration
    D. Occupational Standards for Health Associations

32. An MSDS is used for information on:
    A. patients
    B. phlebotomy technical procedures
    C. chemicals
    D. sharps disposal containers

33. Which of the following is *not* reported as a warning through the NFPA?
    A. fire
    B. chemical instability
    C. PPE
    D. health hazard

34. Chemicals should:
    A. be disposed of in the sink with water gently running
    B. be stored above eye level
    C. be cleaned in a spill with soap and water
    D. be labeled properly

35. When mixing acids and water, you should:
    A. add water to acid
    B. add acid to water
    C. never mix water with acids
    D. add equal amounts in a plastic container

36. Class C fires involve:
    A. gasoline, paints, and/or oil
    B. electrical equipment
    C. wood, paper
    D. flammable materials

37. Patients as well as health care workers may have reactions to latex products that may include:
    A. skin rash
    B. sinus irritation
    C. hives
    D. all of the above

38. The red quadrant of the NFPA rating system indicates what type of hazard?
    A. health hazard
    B. acid or alkali hazard
    C. fire hazard
    D. instability hazard

39. Safety equipment in the chemical area of the health care facility may include:
    A. PPE
    B. emergency shower
    C. eyewash station
    D. all of the above

40. Which of the following are true regarding safety in the health care facility?
    A. Patients' specimens should be covered at all times during transportation.
    B. Always wear required PPE for specimen collections.
    C. Specimen collection trays should be disinfected at least once a week.
    D. All of the above are true

41. Electrical safety involves:
    A. knowing the locations of fire extinguishers in the health care facility
    B. distance, time, and shielding
    C. knowing the location of the circuit breaker box
    D. knowing the MSDS codes

42. Which of the following products do *not* have to be considered in regards to a possible latex hazard to the patient and/or health care worker?
    A. blood pressure cuff
    B. disposable gloves
    C. adhesive tape
    D. all of the above may contain latex

43. If a health care worker has a chemical splashed into his or her eye, the first thing the victim should do is:
    A. Wipe the eye with a sterile gauze.
    B. Run to the emergency room.
    C. Immediately flush the eye with water for 15 minutes.
    D. Call the supervisor within the specimen collection area.

44. Figure 6.1 is a/an:
    A. electrical hazard sign
    B. radiation hazard sign
    C. biohazardous sign
    D. combustible hazard sign

FIGURE 6.1.

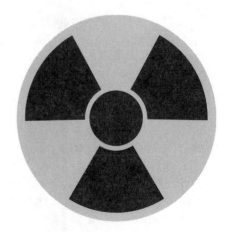

45. To put out a fire in a person's hair or clothes, use
   A. the fire extinguisher for Class D fires
   B. a first aid kit
   C. the fire extinguisher for Class C fires
   D. a fire blanket

46. If acid gets on your skin, wash at once with:
   A. antimicrobial soap
   B. isopropyl alcohol
   C. water
   D. antimicrobial cleanser

47. To be able to put out a fire safely, you should know:
   A. how to use an extinguisher
   B. where the extinguisher is located
   C. how to use a fire blanket
   D. all of the above

48. A bottle of sulfuric acid may be carried through the health care facility in

   A. your hand
   B. your latex-free gloved hand
   C. an acid carrier
   D. a heavy cardboard box

49. The sign shown on the container in Figure 6.2 is a/an:
   A. biohazardous sign
   B. radiation sign
   C. electrical hazard sign
   D. combustible hazard sign

50. If an electrical accident occurs involving electrical shock to an employee or patient, the health care worker should:
   A. shut off the electrical power source
   B. pull the electrocuted person from the electrical source
   C. call medical assistance and start CPR immediately
   D. both A and C

FIGURE 6.2.

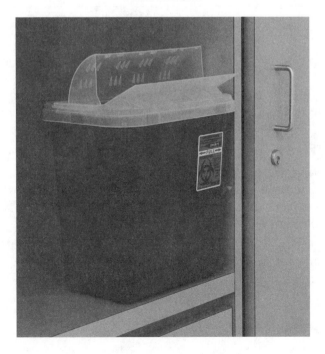

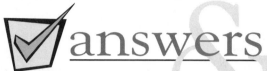

answers & rationales

1.

A. Safe working conditions must be ensured by the employer and have been mandated by law under the Occupational Safety and Health Administration (OSHA) standards. (p. 158)

B, C, D. Safe working conditions must be ensured by the employer and have been mandated by law under OSHA standards.

2.

A. The health care provider will not likely encounter a fire hazard when he or she enters the nuclear medicine department to obtain a blood specimen from a patient.

B. The health care provider is most likely to encounter a radiation hazard when he or she enters the nuclear medicine department to obtain a blood specimen from a patient. (p. 165)

C. The health care provider will not likely encounter a mechanical hazard when he or she enters the nuclear medicine department to obtain a blood specimen from a patient.

D. The health care provider will not likely encounter an electrical hazard when he or she enters the nuclear medicine department to obtain a blood specimen from a patient.

3.

A, C, D. If the fire is small, attempt to extinguish it, using the proper equipment and only after following the first procedural step.

B. If a health care provider is in an area of the health care facility where a fire starts, he or she should *first* pull the lever in the fire alarm box. (p. 159)

4.

A. Needles, syringes, and lancets should be disposed of in a special sturdy container.

B. Gloves should be worn by the phlebotomist for performing blood collection procedures, including transporting various specimens. Latex-free gloves are available for the phlebotomist if he or she is allergic to the latex gloves. (p. 162)

C. The specimen collection area should be disinfected periodically according to the clinical laboratory schedule.

D. The patients' specimens should be covered at all times during transportation.

5.

A. EPA as well as OSHA, state, and local regulations and laws regulate the disposal of waste. (p. 161)

B. The Clinical Laboratory Standards Institute (CLSI), formerly NCCLS, provides standards for disposal of biological and chemical wastes but does not actually regulate waste disposal.

C. The National Fire Protection Association (NFPA) oversees fire safety, not biological waste disposal.

D. The Joint Commission on Accreditation of Healthcare Organizations provides accrediting standards for disposal of biological waste but does not regulate biological waste disposal.

6.

A. Sending for medical assistance should be the second step in controlling severe bleeding.

B. Starting cardiopulmonary resuscitation (CPR) should occur if the person's breathing movements stop or the person's lips, tongue, and fingernails become blue.

C. The first step in controlling severe bleeding is to apply pressure directly over the wound or venipuncture site. (pp. 174–175)

D. The first step in controlling severe bleeding is to apply pressure directly over the wound or venipuncture site.

7.

A. If a health care provider is caught in a fire in the health care institution, he or she should *not* run. (p. 159)

B. If a health care provider is caught in a fire in the health care institution, he or she should close all doors and windows before leaving the area.

C. If a health care provider is caught in a fire in the health care institution, he or she should attempt to extinguish the fire if it is small.

D. If a health care provider is caught in a fire in the health care institution, he or she should call the assigned fire number.

8.

A. The victim of a chemical accident must not rub the affected area vigorously.

B. The victim of a chemical accident must immediately rinse the affected area with water for at least 15 minutes after removing contaminated clothing.

C. The victim of a chemical accident must not immediately rinse the affected area with a neutral chemical.

D. The victim of a chemical accident must immediately rinse the affected area with water for at least 15 minutes after removing contaminated clothing. (p. 168)

9.

A, B, C. Any explosive flammables must be stored in an explosion-proof or fireproof room or cabinet.

D. Any explosive flammables must be stored in an explosion-proof or fireproof room or cabinet. (p. 169)

10.

A. The yellow quadrant of the NFPA's 0 to 4 hazard rating system does not indicate a flammability hazard.

B. The yellow quadrant of the NFPA's 0 to 4 hazard rating system does not indicate a health hazard.

C. The yellow quadrant of the NFPA's 0 to 4 hazard rating system indicates an instability hazard. (p. 168)

D. The yellow quadrant of the NFPA's 0 to 4 hazard rating system does not indicate a specific hazard.

11.

A. The blue quadrant of the NFPA's 0 to 4 hazard rating system does not indicate a flammability hazard.

B. The blue quadrant of the NFPA's 0 to 4 hazard rating system indicates a health hazard. (p. 168)

C. The blue quadrant of the NFPA's 0 to 4 hazard rating system does not indicate an instability hazard.

D. The blue quadrant of the NFPA's 0 to 4 hazard rating system does not indicate a specific hazard.

12.

A. If an electrical accident occurs involving electrical shock for an employee or a patient, the *first* thing that the health care worker should do is "not" to move the victim.

B. If an electrical accident occurs involving electrical shock for an employee or a patient, the *first* thing that the health care worker should do is shut off electrical power. (p. 164)

C. Medical assistance should be called and cardiopulmonary resuscitation (CPR) started immediately *after* the electrical power is shut off.

D. A blanket should be placed over the electrocuted victim after the electrical power is shut off.

13.

A, C, D. The three cardinal principles of self-protection from radiation exposure are time, shielding, and distance.

B. The three cardinal principles of self-protection from radiation exposure are time, shielding, and distance. (p. 164)

14.

A. OSHA amended the Hazard Communication Standard (29 CFR 1910.1200) to include health care facilities. Thus labels for hazardous chemicals must (1) provide a warning (e.g., corrosive), (2) explain the nature of the hazard, (3) state special precautions to eliminate risks, and (4) explain first-aid treatment in the event of a leak, a chemical spill, or other exposure to the chemical. (pp. 166–167)

B. The EPA does not oversee MSDSs.

C. NFPA does not oversee MSDSs.

D. CDC does not oversee MSDSs.

15.

A. Opening the airway by checking for obstructions is the third step in giving mouth-to-mouth resuscitation. The first step in giving mouth-to-mouth resuscitation is to determine whether the victim is conscious by gently shaking the victim and yelling, "Are you okay?"

B. The first step in giving mouth-to-mouth resuscitation is to determine whether the victim is conscious by gently shaking the victim and yelling, "Are you okay?"

C. The first step in giving mouth-to-mouth resuscitation is to determine whether the victim is conscious by gently shaking the victim and yelling, "Are you okay?" (p. 176)

D. The first step in giving mouth-to-mouth resuscitation is to determine whether the victim is conscious by gently shaking the victim and yelling, "Are you okay?"

16.

A. For chemical safety in a health care facility, no chemicals should be stored above eye level because of the danger of breakage involved when reaching.

B. It is advisable to wear an apron over the laboratory coat for additional protection against chemical burns.

C. An acid carrier should be used when transporting alkalis or acids. (p. 169)

D. All explosives should be stored in an exposion-proof room.

17.

A. Fluids should not be given to a shock victim since they may require surgery or a general anesthetic.

B. The shock victim should be kept warm.

C. The shock victim should be kept in a lying position. (p. 177)

D. For a shock victim, elevate the victim's legs so that the head is lower than the trunk.

18.

A, B, C. OSHA requires adherence to Standard Precautions when health care workers respond to emergencies that provide potential exposure to blood.

D. OSHA requires adherence to Standard Precautions when health care workers respond to emergencies that provide potential exposure to blood. (p. 175)

19.

A, C, D. If blood has been spilled, wear gloves and use a 1:10 bleach solution or commercially prepared solution to clean the area. Keep the bleach in contact with the contaminated area for a minimum of 20 minutes.

B. If blood has been spilled, wear gloves and use a 1:10 bleach solution or commercially prepared solution to clean the area. Keep the bleach in contact with the contaminated area for a minimum of 20 minutes. (p. 162)

20.

A. If an accidental needlestick injury occurs to a phlebotomist, CBC and hemoglobin tests may be performed but are not mandatory.

B. If an accidental needlestick injury occurs to a phlebotomist, he or she should be counseled and evaluated for HIV and HCV at periodic intervals. (p. 162)

C. If an accidental needlestick injury occurs to a phlebotomist, blood pH test is usually not performed.

D. If an accidental needlestick injury occurs to a phlebotomist, he or she should be counseled and evaluated for HIV and HCV at periodic intervals.

21.

A. MSDS is not an abbreviation for Material Serum Data Sheets.

B. MSDS is not an abbreviation for Material Safety Drug Sheets.

C. MSDS is an abbreviation for Material Safety Data Sheets. (p. 166)

D. MSDS is not an abbreviation for Material Serum Drug Sheets.

22.

A. The FDA did not develop a labeling system for hazardous chemicals that is frequently used in health care facilities.

B. The NFPA (National Fire Protection Association) developed a labeling system for hazardous chemicals that is frequently used in health care facilities. (p. 167)

C. The CDC did not develop a labeling system for hazardous chemicals that is frequently used in health care facilities.

D. The CLSI did not develop a labeling system for hazardous chemicals that is frequently used in health care facilities.

23.

A, B, D. The phlebotomist needs at least two patient identifiers, neither of which can be the patient's room number or patient's location when collecting blood specimens.

C. The phlebotomist needs at least two patient identifiers, neither of which can be the patient's room number or patient's location when collecting blood specimens. (p. 171)

24.

A. Gloves are a PPE that may or may not be made of latex and must be checked prior to use in a latex-safe environment.

B. A laboratory coat is a PPE that is not made of latex and can be used without latex precautions. (p. 173)

C. Tourniquets must be checked to see if they are made of latex.

D. Syringes must be checked to see if they are made of latex.

25.

A, C, D. For Class A fires, you can use pressurized water and/or dry chemical fire extinguishers.

B. For Class A fires, you can use pressurized water and/or dry chemical fire extinguishers. (p. 160)

26.

A. The chemicals with a blue storage code does not indicate they are highly corrosive.

B. The chemicals with a blue storage code does not indicate they may detonate.

C. The chemicals with a blue storage code indicate they are a health hazard. (p. 168)

D. The chemicals with a blue storage code does not indicate they are flammable.

27.

A, C, D. A tourniquet should not be used to control bleeding in an emergency except in the case of an amputated, mangled, or crushed arm or leg or for profuse bleeding that cannot be stopped otherwise.

B. A tourniquet should not be used to control bleeding in an emergency except in the case of an amputated, mangled, or crushed arm or leg or for profuse bleeding that cannot be stopped otherwise. (p. 175)

28.

A. A fire that occurs in or near electrical equipment is not a Class A fire.

B. A fire that occurs in or near electrical equipment is not a Class B fire.

C. A fire that occurs in or near electrical equipment is a Class C fire. (p. 160)

D. A fire that occurs in or near electrical equipment is not a Class D fire.

29.

A. A solution of bleach used for cleaning the specimen collection area should not be at a concentration of 1:1.

B. A solution of bleach used for cleaning the specimen collection area should not be at a concentration of 1:2.

C. A solution of bleach used for cleaning the specimen collection area should be at a concentration of 1:10. (p. 162)

D. A solution of bleach used for cleaning the specimen collection area should not be at a concentration of 1:20.

30.

A, C, D. When using a fire extinguisher, the operator should try to remember the acronym PASS for *P*ull pin; *A*im nozzle; *S*queeze handle; *S*weep side to side.

B. When using a fire extinguisher, the operator should try to remember the acronym PASS for *P*ull pin; *A*im nozzle; *S*queeze handle; *S*weep side to side. (p. 160)

31.

A. OSHA does not stand for Occupational Standards and Health Administration.

B. OSHA stands for Occupational Safety and Health Administration. (p. 158)

C. OSHA does not stand for Occupational Safety and Hazards Administration.

D. OSHA does not stand for Occupational Standards for Health Associations.

32.

A, B, D. Material Safety Data Sheets (MSDSs) are required for any chemicals with a hazard warning label.

C. Material Safety Data Sheets (MSDSs) are required for any chemicals with a hazard warning label. (pp. 166–167)

33.

A, B, D. The National Fire Protection Association (NFPA) provides warning information for fires and a labeling system for hazardous chemicals, but does not oversee personal protection equipment (PPE).

C. The National Fire Protection Association (NFPA) provides warning information for fires and a labeling system for hazardous chemicals, but does not oversee personal protection equipment (PPE). (pp. 158, 160, 166)

34.

A. Chemicals should not be disposed of in the sink, but rather disposed of in the manner required through the local and state regulations.

B. No chemicals should be stored above eye level because of the danger of breakage involved in reaching.

C. If a chemical spill occurs, the health care worker should obtain a spill cleanup kit from the clinical chemistry section. The kit includes absorbents and neutralizers to clean up acids, alkalis, and other chemicals.

D. All chemicals must be labeled properly since they pose health and/or physical hazards. (pp. 166–167)

35.

A, C, D. ALWAYS add acid to water. NEVER add water to acid.

B. ALWAYS add acid to water. NEVER add water to acid. (p. 166)

36.

A. Class C fires do not involve gasoline, paints, and/or oils.

B. Class C fires involve electrical equipment. (p. 160)

C. Class C fires do not involve wood or paper.

D. Class C fires involve electrical equipment.

37.

A, B, C. Patients as well as health care workers may have allergic reactions to latex products (i.e., gloves, syringes, tourniquets, etc.) that include skin rashes, hives, sinus irritation, and, sometimes, shock.

D. Patients as well as health care workers may have allergic reactions to latex products (i.e., gloves, syringes, tourniquets, etc.) that include skin rashes, hives, sinus irritation, and, sometimes, shock. (pp. 172–173)

38.

A. The red quadrant of the NFPA rating system does not indicate a health hazard.

B. The red quadrant of the NFPA rating system does not indicate an acid or alkali hazard.

C. The red quadrant of the NFPA rating system indicates a fire hazard. (p. 168)

D. The red quadrant of the NFPA rating system does not indicate an instability hazard.

39.

A, B, C. Safety equipment maintained in the chemical area of the health care facility may include personal protective equipment (PPE), an emergency shower, chemical spill cleanup kits, and eyewash stations.

D. Safety equipment maintained in the chemical area of the health care facility may include personal protective equipment (PPE), an emergency shower, chemical spill cleanup kits and eyewash stations. (pp. 166–168)

40.

A, B, C. Safety rules in the health care facility and clinical laboratory include: (1) patients' specimens should be covered at all times during transportation and centrifugation; (2) specimen collection trays must be disinfected at least once a week; and (3) the phlebotomist needs to always wear PPE for specimen collections.

D. Safety rules in the health care facility and clinical laboratory include: (1) patients' specimens should be covered at all times during transportation and centrifugation; (2) specimen collection trays must be disinfected at least once a week; and (3) the phlebotomist needs to always wear PPE for specimen collections. (p. 161)

41.

A. Electrical safety in the health care facility does not involve knowing the location of the fire extinguishers, that is fire safety.

B. Electrical safety in the health care facility does not involve distance, time, and shielding.

C. Electrical safety in the health care facility involves knowing the location of the circuit breaker box. (p. 163)

D. Electrical safety in the health care facility does not involve knowing the MSDS.

42.

A, B, C. Blood pressure cuffs, disposable gloves, and adhesive tape may all contain latex.

D. Blood pressure cuffs, disposable gloves, and adhesive tape may all contain latex. (p. 173)

43.

A. If a health care worker has a chemical splashed into his or her eye, the victim should not wipe the eye.

B. If a health care worker has a chemical splashed into his or her eye, the victim should rinse his or her eyes at the eyewash station for a minimum of 15 minutes.

C. If a health care worker has a chemical splashed into his or her eye, the victim should rinse his or her eye at the eyewash station for a minimum of 15 minutes. (p. 168)

D. If a health care worker has a chemical splashed into his or her eye, the victim should immediately rinse his or her eye at the eyewash station for a minimum of 15 minutes and then call the supervisor.

44.

A. Figure 6.1 does not identify an electrical hazard.

B. Figure 6.1 identifies a radiation hazard. (p. 165)

C. Figure 6.1 does not identify a biohazard.

D. Figure 6.1 does not identify a combustible hazard.

FIGURE 6.1. Radiation hazard sign.

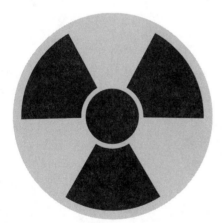

45.

A, B, C. The fire blanket should be used to smother burning clothes, hair, etc., on a person.

D. The fire blanket should be used to smother burning clothes, hair, etc., on a person. (p. 158)

46.

A. If acid gets on your skin, do not rinse immediately with antimicrobial soap.

B. If acid gets on your skin, do not rinse immediately with isopropyl alcohol.

C. If acid gets on your skin, rinse immediately with large amounts of water. (p. 168)

D. If acid gets on your skin, do not rinse immediately with antimicrobial cleanser.

47.

A, B, C. To be able to put out a fire safely, you should know how to use the fire extinguisher, where the fire extinguisher is located, and how to use a fire blanket.

D. To be able to put out a fire safely, you should know how to use the fire extinguisher, where the fire extinguisher is located and how to use a fire blanket. (p. 158)

48.

A. A bottle of sulfuric acid must not be carried through the health care facility in your hand.

B. A bottle of sulfuric acid must not be carried through the health care facility in your hand.

C. A bottle of sulfuric acid may be carried through the health care facility in an acid carrier. (p. 169)

D. A bottle of sulfuric acid must not be carried through the health care facility in a cardboard box.

49.

A. Figure 6.2 has a biohazardous sign on the sharps container. (p. 162)

B. Figure 6.2 does not have a radiation sign on the sharps container.

C. Figure 6.2 does not have an electrical hazard sign on the sharps container.

D. Figure 6.2 does not have a combustible hazard sign on the sharps container.

FIGURE 6.2. Sharps container.

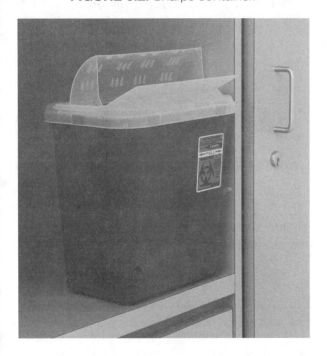

50.

A, B, C. If an electrical accident has occurred involving electrical shock to an employee or a patient, the health care worker should shut off the electrical power and call for medical assistance and immediately start CPR.

D. If an electrical accident has occurred involving electrical shock to an employee or a patient, the health care worker should shut off the electrical power and call for medical assistance and immediately start CPR. (p. 164)

7 Documentation, Specimen Handling, and Transportation

chapter objectives

Upon completion of Chapter 7, the learner is responsible for the following:

➤ Describe the basic components and uses of a medical record.

➤ Describe acceptable guidelines for maintaining privacy and confidentiality.

➤ Describe essential elements of requisition and report forms.

➤ Name three methods commonly used to transport specimens.

DIRECTIONS Each of the questions or incomplete statements below is followed by four suggested answers or completions. Select one answer that is best in each case.

1. Why is documentation of all clinical events important?
   A. To monitor quality and coordination of care.
   B. So that only the patient's physician can access the information.
   C. So that employees can get merit raises.
   D. So public information may be disclosed during a financial inquiry.

2. A nurse stated to a phlebotomist that one of a patient's lab test results was a mistake. The nurse asked the phlebotomist to change the test result immediately. What should the phlebotomist do?
   A. make the change immediately
   B. investigate the situation more thoroughly prior to taking action
   C. leave the test result as it is
   D. call OSHA

3. When documenting errors in a medical record, which of the following statements is most appropriate?
   A. Errors should be erased or deleted.
   B. Errors should be reported to the local newspaper.
   C. The phlebotomist should give her opinion about who made the mistake.
   D. Errors should not be erased, but noted and corrected.

4. The phlebotomist has the greatest impact on which phase of laboratory testing?
   A. post-analytic phase
   B. preanalytic phase

C. analytic phase
D. specimen processing

5. Which of the following variables represents a preanalytic variable that might affect laboratory testing results?
   A. not wearing a laboratory coat
   B. reporting laboratory test results to the nurse
   C. the patient ate a hearty breakfast
   D. the specimen is tested on a calibrated instrument

6. If a phlebotomist wanted to look up specimen tube requirements while on duty at her hospital, what would probably be the best source for the information?
   A. infection control procedures
   B. QC procedures
   C. call a friend who works at a similar hospital to see what they use
   D. specimen collection manual

7. Like many laboratory departments, one hospital's policies did not allow release of information directly to patients. However, a patient made an emergency telephone call to the laboratory and asked a specific question about her own laboratory result. What was the most appropriate course of action for the phlebotomist?
   A. Using a professional tone of voice, provide the patient with the information requested.
   B. Using a professional tone of voice, follow the organization's directions

about referring the patient to the appropriate person.

C. Provide a detailed explanation of the reasons for the policy and report the situation to a supervisor.

D. Place the caller on hold while seeking an exception to the rule.

8. A phlebotomist inadvertently overheard a conversation between a doctor and a patient about a medical condition that is unrelated to the specimen collection or laboratory testing process. What is the best course of action regarding the sharing of this information with other individuals in the hospital?

A. The information can be shared since it was already shared with the doctor.

B. The information is privileged and should not be shared.

C. The information is medically related and can be shared with anyone in the hospital.

D. The information is classified and should not be shared.

9. Identify one trait found in a "privacy-conscious" organization?

A. Strict security measures are in place.

B. The organization informs patients about use and disclosure of medical information.

C. Only medical information is disclosed.

D. The organization is not-for-profit.

10. A phlebotomist was asked by a patient to fax test results to her home so she would not have to go back to the doctor. What is the most appropriate course of action for the phlebotomist?

A. Follow the employer's policies regarding the use or transmission of lab results.

B. Fax the test results the first time only.

C. Refuse to fax the test results, but give the patient a verbal report.

D. Fax the test results under the condition that the patient must return to her doctor.

11. Bar codes can be used in health care for patient identification purposes. Which of the following characterizes how bar codes are interpreted?

A. The bars indicate pricing for laboratory procedures.

B. Light and dark bands of varying widths represent alphanumeric symbols.

C. They contain the name of the institution.

D. They reveal the nature of each specimen.

12. The most efficient and accurate way of making labels for specimens is by:

A. imprinting the physician's orders directly from a card file

B. printing from a computerized system

C. manually labeling the specimens as each one is drawn

D. prelabel all the tubes to be collected for the day

13. What is a "RFID"?

A. blood test for rheumatoid factor

B. urine test that must be transported on ice

C. test code for a rapid screening test

D. identification tag using silicon chips and a wireless receiver

14. What type of information *cannot* be converted into bar code symbols?

A. supplies and equipment inventory

B. laboratory test codes

C. handwritten information

D. date of patient's birth

15. A phlebotomist noticed that new printed labels for laboratory specimens came with a smaller transfer label. What could this smaller label be used for?
    A. aliquot tubes, cuvettes, microscope slides
    B. bandage for patient's finger
    C. medical record file
    D. chemical reagents

16. Serum should be transported to the laboratory for testing and separated from blood cells within which of the following time periods to prevent erroneous test results?
    A. 5 hours
    B. 4 hours
    C. 2 hours
    D. 5 minutes

17. Which of the following organizations provides standards for handling and processing blood specimens?
    A. CED
    B. CDC
    C. NCA
    D. CLSI

18. Approximately how long does it take a normal blood specimen to clot?
    A. 1–2 minutes
    B. 5–15 minutes
    C. 30–60 minutes
    D. over 2 hours

19. The term "thermolabile" refers to a trait of some chemical constituents that are tested in blood specimens. What does it mean?
    A. constituents are affected by temperature
    B. constituents are affected by light
    C. constituents are affected by the method of draw
    D. constituents are affected by the time of day that the specimen is drawn

20. Excessive agitation of a specimen is likely to cause which of the following conditions?
    A. thorough mixing of the anticoagulant with the blood
    B. warming of the specimen
    C. chilling of the specimen
    D. hemolysis in the specimen

21. Some specimens must be wrapped in aluminum foil during transportation. What purpose does this serve?
    A. keeps the specimen warm
    B. keeps the specimen cool
    C. protects the specimen from light
    D. protects the specimen from unnecessary agitation

22. Hemolyzed specimens cause which of the following?
    A. chemical interference with lab assays
    B. warming of the specimen
    C. cooling of the specimen
    D. centrifugation interference

23. If a blood specimen has a separation device, how many times should it be centrifuged?
    A. maximum of 8 times
    B. 5–7 times
    C. 2–4 times
    D. 1 time

24. If the laboratory must save serum or plasma for testing later, how would most specimens be stored?
    A. indefinitely at room temperature
    B. indefinitely in a refrigerator
    C. in the frost-free frozen section of a refrigerator
    D. in a freezer at or below −20 degrees C

25. Glycolytic action refers to what condition?
    A. lysing of the red blood cells
    B. lysing of the white blood cells
    C. breakdown of glucose
    D. platelet activation

26. Why should one use an airtight container with icy water to transport an arterial specimen for blood gas analysis?
    A. It decreases the loss of gases from the specimen.
    B. It promotes coagulation.
    C. It aids in the instrumentation phase of the testing process.
    D. It increases the oxygen content in the specimen.

27. Assays that require a chilled specimen include all but which one?
    A. gastrin, ammonia, and lactic acid
    B. renin, catecholamine, and parathyroid hormone determinations
    C. blood gases
    D. blood cultures

28. To chill a blood specimen as it is transported, the health care worker should use:
    A. tepid water
    B. a small freezer unit
    C. icy water
    D. frozen blocks of ice

29. Specimens that require protection from light include those for:
    A. CBC, diff, and platelet counts
    B. PT and PTTs
    C. bilirubin and some vitamins
    D. none of the above

30. Specimens that require warming to body temperature are those for:

A. CBC, diff, and platelet counts
B. PT and PTTs
C. bilirubin and some vitamins
D. cold agglutinins and cryofibrinogen

31. Most laboratories require that primary specimen tubes be placed in which of the following during transportation?
    A. biohazard box
    B. leakproof plastic bag
    C. aluminum foil
    D. icy water

32. Why should blood and urine specimens for microbiological culture be transported to the laboratory quickly?
    A. So that blood cells will not rupture.
    B. To improve the likelihood of detecting pathogens.
    C. To keep the specimens close to body temperature.
    D. To avoid excessive exposure to light

33. One of the most efficient and safe methods of specimen transportation in a large health care organization is:
    A. hand-carrying the specimen
    B. clear biohazard carts
    C. pneumatic tube systems
    D. email for specimens

34. Laboratory reports containing test results should go through which of the following protocols?
    A. Release results immediately upon completion of the testing process.
    B. Confirm results, date the release of results, and send a permanent copy to the clinical record.
    C. Call the results to a physician.
    D. Fax the results immediately to the patient.

35. Specimens for diagnostic testing other than blood may need to be transported by health care workers using special handling procedures. In a hospital clinical laboratory department, these specimens would usually *not* include:
    A. crime scene artifacts
    B. body fluids
    C. tissues
    D. blood components

36. In designing a report form for laboratory results, which one of the listed elements is not required?
    A. patient and physician identification
    B. date and time of collection
    C. reference ranges
    D. patient and physician addresses

37. The use of a blood drawing list or log sheet in a specimen collection area serves to:
    A. provide a record of specimens collected
    B. keep confidential information available
    C. keep track of employee productivity
    D. track quality control of supplies/reagents

38. Which of the following factors would *not* be considered when using pneumatic tube systems for transporting specimens?
    A. mechanical reliability and distance of transport
    B. speed of carrier and landing mechanism
    C. effect on the chemical and cellular components of specimens
    D. quality control of supplies

39. The most reliable labeling method for avoiding transcription errors in specimen collection is:
    A. handwritten labels with careful attention to detail

B. computerized labels using bar codes
C. addressograph machine
D. prelabeling specimen tubes at the beginning of a work shift

40. Quality control records do *not* include information about:
    A. employee health
    B. proper use and storage information
    C. expiration dates and stability information
    D. precision and accuracy of testing supplies/reagents

41. Bar codes in phlebotomy applications can be used for all but which one?
    A. patient's arm preference
    B. specimen accession numbers, test codes
    C. product numbers, inventory expiration dates
    D. patient names, DOB, patient identification numbers

42. Preanalytical errors include transportation variables. One example is:
    A. breakage in the pneumatic tube
    B. inadequate centrifugation
    C. inadequate volume in the test tube
    D. patient stress and anxiety

43. Preanalytical errors include patient variables. One example is:
    A. tube breakage
    B. inadequate centrifugation
    C. inadequate volume in the test tube
    D. patient stress and anxiety

44. Preanalytical errors include specimen processing variables. Which variable would not be part of specimen processing?
    A. excessive shaking or mixing
    B. inadequate centrifugation

C. exposure to heat or light

D. analytic instrumentation malfunction

45. Another name often used for a "critical value" is:

A. radical value

B. random value

C. panic value

D. static value

Questions 46–48 relate to the following case scenario:

Marie was a medical assistant in a family health clinic with a small laboratory. She had responsibilities in several areas, including answering the phone in the laboratory, drawing blood specimens, clerical duties, and assisting with laboratory testing. One morning when the clinic was particularly busy, she was drawing blood for numerous patients and trying to process them so that they could be tested in a timely manner. When the phone rang, she was reluctant to answer it because she had almost finished processing a batch of samples. It rang several times; then she hurried to pick it up and asked the individual to "hold please." She went back to finish processing the samples and forgot the person on hold. Later, she found out that the individual on hold was a doctor who was trying to request another test on a previously drawn sample.

46. What should Mary have said when she first answered the phone?

A. "Hold for just a moment, please."

B. "Please hold while I process a few specimens so that they will not be delayed."

C. "Hello, this is the clinic laboratory. May I help you?"

D. "Hello, I am sorry that I cannot assist you now. Please call back."

47. Additional training would benefit Mary. Which of the following topics would be the *lowest* priority for her continuing education?

A. customer service and time management

B. centrifugation basics

C. communication

D. placing a caller on hold and phone technology

48. To improve communication and enhance the flow of information in a hospital setting, which type of technology would be *least* helpful to assist the laboratory in the processing of specimens?

A. satellite radio

B. a fax machine for receiving requests

C. barcoding specimens

D. speakerphone

Questions 49–50 relate to the following case scenario:

A medical technician working in a large academic hospital laboratory was asked to package and send several serum specimens to a research laboratory in Switzerland. She knew that many of the doctors were working on research in collaboration with scientists in other countries. She vaguely remembered that there were special procedures for this request but she did not know what they were. She realized that there were serious fines and legal implications if she did not comply with the procedures.

49. Which of the following is *not* the employer's responsibility in complying with this request?

A. provide information and training

B. negotiating arrangements for package carriers of the specimens

C. providing security through customs

D. acquiring confirmation of delivery

50. Which of the following is *not* the employee's responsibility in complying with this request?
    A. prepare primary and secondary containers
    B. identify, classify, pack, mark, label specimens
    C. notify carrier of shipping details and confirm delivery
    D. contact customs agents about the specimens

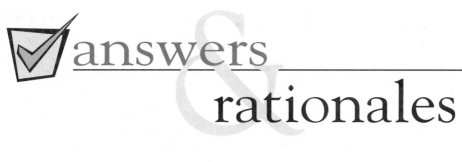

answers & rationales

1.

A. Documentation of all clinical events is important for monitoring the quality of care given to the patient, for coordination of care among members of the health care team, to comply with accrediting and licensing standards, to provide legal protection, and in some cases for research purposes. (pp. 182–183)

B. The medical record is a legal document that is available not only to the patient's physician, but also to other members of the patient's health care team. Documentation in the medical record provides proof of the quality of care given.

C. The medical record may include documentation if errors are made; however, it is not usually the only documentation required if an employee is being terminated.

D. The medical record is a confidential, private record and is not subject to review by the general public. Information may not be disclosed during a financial inquiry unless the hospital or patient gives permission.

2.

A. The phlebotomist should *not* make the change immediately.

B. Records should never be changed or altered to cover a mistake. Errors should be noted according to the institution's policies. Generally speaking, the phlebotomist should investigate the situation more thoroughly prior to taking action. It should be reported to a supervisor to identify causes for the mistake (if it really is one) and to take all corrective actions. (pp. 182–183)

C. The phlebotomist should investigate the situation thoroughly and defer the decision to a supervisor rather than leaving the test result as it is without further action.

D. This situation does not warrant a call to OSHA. It is not the type of problem they investigate.

3.

A. Errors should never be erased or deleted.

B. Errors should not be reported to the local newspaper

C. The phlebotomist should not give her opinion about who is to blame; rather, only the facts should be recorded in these situations.

D. When documenting errors in a medical record, errors should never be erased or deleted. They should be noted in a special manner along with the corrected information. (pp. 182–183)

4.

A. The post-analytic phase of laboratory testing usually refers to the period after the specimen has been analyzed; this is when test results are reported.

B. The phlebotomist has the greatest impact on the preanalytic phase of laboratory testing. (p. 184)

C. The analytic phase refers to the testing processes.

D. Specimen processing occurs during the preanalytic phase, but there are also other responsibilities that are impacted by the phlebotomist in this phase, that is, technique, transportation, etc.

5.

A. Failure to wear a laboratory coat will not have an effect on laboratory testing results, but the use of appropriate protective equipment and supplies such as a laboratory coat or jacket is recommended for safety and hygiene reasons.

B. Reporting laboratory test results to the nurse would not have an effect on laboratory results because it is part of the post-analytic process.

C. The fact that a patient ate a hearty breakfast represents a preanalytic variable that will likely affect laboratory testing results. (pp. 183–184)

D. The fact that a specimen is tested on a calibrated instrument does not have an effect on preanalytic variables. It should not have an adverse effect on laboratory results because it is part of the analytic process in a normal testing situation.

6.

A. Infection control manuals relate to procedures designed to prevent the spread of infections in the health care environment (e.g., precautions, isolation procedures, disposal, and decontamination methods). These manuals do not usually contain specimen tube requirements.

B. Quality control (QC) procedures relate to maintaining stability and monitoring supplies,

reagents, and equipment, and measuring precision and accuracy of testing processes. QC manuals do not usually contain specimen tube requirements.

C. Calling a coworker to inquire about specimen tube requirements is not usually the best method to ascertain specimen tube requirements.

D. Specimen collection manuals, either electronic or paper versions, contain information about patient preparation, specimen tube requirements, timing requirements, preservative and anticoagulants, special handling or transportation needs, and clinical information needed for specific tests. (p. 186)

7.

A. Health care organizations have strict policies and procedures about releasing patient information. The phlebotomist should never release information unless authorized to do so. In this case, the phlebotomist was not authorized to release information directly to the patient.

B. In this case, the phlebotomist was justified in politely and professionally referring the patient to an appropriate person who is authorized to counsel the patient and/or provide the requested information. (pp. 185, 188)

C. A policy discussion that does not directly relate to the health care worker's role in caring for the patient should be avoided.

D. Placing the caller on hold is appropriate for short-term periods of time. In this scenario, the period on hold would likely be lengthy so it is not advisable.

8.

A. Patient information should not be shared with individuals who are not directly involved in the care of a patient without the prior consent of the patient.

B. Patient information should not be shared with individuals who are not directly involved

in the care of a patient without the prior consent of the patient. In this case, the communication that was overheard is considered privileged and private. (p. 188)

C. Patient information should not be shared with individuals who are not directly involved in the care of a patient without the prior consent of the patient.

D. The patient information presented in this case is considered private and confidential, not "classified." Patient information should not be shared with individuals who are not directly involved in the care of a patient without the prior consent of the patient.

9.

A. "Strict security measures" implies protocols and methods to keep the organization safe.

B. "Privacy-conscious" organizations inform patients about the use and disclosure of their health information and require that only the minimum amount of health information be disclosed when necessary. (p. 188)

C. The statement "only medical information is disclosed" is not a trait of a "privacy-conscious" organization.

D. Being a "not-for-profit" organization relates to the financial structure and is not a trait of a privacy-conscious organization.

10.

A through D. (Correct answer is A.) HIPAA laws apply to fax transmissions even though the use of electronic transmissions is a timely way of communicating. However, patients' permissions are needed to disclose information and each facility should have policies related to the use of electronic transmissions. (p. 188)

11.

A. When describing bar code usage for patient identification purposes, they do not typically indicate pricing.

B. When describing bar code usage for patient identification purposes, they are interpreted by using light and dark bands of varying widths that represent alphanumeric symbols (i.e., a name and number). (p. 189)

C. When describing bar code usage for patient identification purposes, they do not usually contain the name of the institution.

D. When describing bar code usage for patient identification purposes, they do not usually reveal the type of specimen.

12.

A. Imprinting the physician's orders directly from the card file is not the most accurate or efficient method of labeling specimens.

B. The most accurate method to generate specimen labels is by using computerized systems. Computerization of the collection process can significantly decrease errors because data are continually being checked against the computer files, and authorized individuals can add to and receive designated information. (p. 191)

C. Manually labeling the specimens as each one is drawn is not as accurate or efficient as using computer-generated labels because it is prone to transcription errors.

D. Prelabeling all the specimen tubes is not recommended due to the potential for mix-ups.

13.

A. RFID is not a test for rheumatoid factor.

B. RFID is not a urine test.

C. RFID is not a test code for a rapid screening test.

D. RFID, radio frequency identification, is another form of identification tag that is used for identifying and tracking records, specimens, patients, equipment, and supplies. It uses a silicon chip that transmits data to a wireless receiver. (p. 189)

14.

A. Supplies and equipment inventory can be barcoded.

B. Laboratory test codes can be barcoded

C. Handwritten information cannot be directly barcoded. (p. 191)

D. Patients' birthdates can be barcoded.

15.

A. Small printed transfer labels can be used for aliquot tubes, cuvettes, and microscope slides. (p. 193)

B. Small printed transfer labels cannot be used to bandage a patient's finger.

C. Small printed transfer labels are not normally used in the medical record.

D. Small printed transfer labels are not normally used for chemical reagents.

16.

A. Five hours would result in excessive delays after blood collection, resulting in glycolytic action from the blood cells interfering with the analysis of several constituents, including glucose.

B. Four hours would also result in excessive delays after blood collection, resulting in glycolytic action from the blood cells interfering with the analysis of several constituents, including glucose.

C. Blood specimens should always be transported to the clinical laboratory for testing as soon as possible, ideally within 45 minutes but no more than 2 hours from the time of collection so that the serum or plasma can be separated from the blood cells. Once separated, serum may remain at room temperature, be refrigerated, be stored in a dark place, or be frozen, depending on the test methodology. Serum should be covered to prevent evapora-

tion, which can cause some constituents to become more concentrated and thus cause erroneous results. (pp. 194–195)

D. Five minutes is not enough time to allow the blood to clot adequately and is usually not a realistic transport time for most clinical specimens, with the exception of a laboratory located at the site of collection or a point-of-service scenario.

17.

A. CED does *not* represent an organization for laboratory standards.

B. JCAHO, the Joint Commission for Accreditation of Health Care Organizations, does *not* provide standards for handling blood specimens.

C. NCA, National Credentialing Agency for Laboratory Personnel, does *not* provide standards for handling and processing blood specimens.

D. The Clinical Laboratory Standards Institute, CLSI, formerly known as the National Committee for Clinical Laboratory Standards, provides standards for handling and processing blood specimens. (pp. 194–195)

18.

A. It takes longer than 1–2 minutes for a blood specimen to clot.

B. It takes longer than 5–15 minutes for a blood specimen to clot.

C. It takes approximately 30–60 minutes for a normal blood specimen to clot. (pp. 194–195)

D. It does not normally take over 2 hours for a normal blood specimen to clot.

19.

A. The term "thermolabile" refers to chemical constituents that are affected by temperature. (pp. 194–195)

B. The term "light sensitive" refers to chemical constituents that are affected by light.

C and D. The term "thermolabile" refers to chemical constituents that are affected by temperature, not by the method of draw by the time of day that the specimen is drawn.

20.

A. Excessive agitation of a specimen will cause thorough mixing of the anticoagulant with the blood, but is not recommended due to the possibility of hemolysis.

B. Excessive agitation of a specimen is not likely to cause warming of the specimen.

C. Excessive agitation of a specimen will not cause chilling of the specimen.

D. Excessive agitation of a specimen is likely to cause hemolysis in the specimen. (pp. 194–195)

21.

A and B. Wrapping specimens in aluminum foil during transportation protects them from light; it does not serve to keep the specimen warm or cool.

C. Wrapping specimens in aluminum foil during transportation protects them from light. (p. 195)

D. Wrapping specimens in aluminum foil during transportation protects them from light; it does not serve to keep the specimen from unnecessary agitation.

22.

A. Hemolyzed specimens cause chemical interference with lab assays. (p. 194)

B and C. Hemolyzed specimens cause chemical interference with lab assays, *not* warming or cooling of the specimens.

D. Hemolyzed specimens cause chemical interference with lab assays, *not* centrifugation interference.

23.

A, B, C. A specimen should not be centrifuged more than once, *not* "a maximum of 8 times," "5–7 times," or "2–4 times."

D. A specimen should not be centrifuged more than once. (p. 195)

24.

A, B, C. If the laboratory must save serum or plasma for testing later, it should *not* be stored indefinitely at room temperature, stored indefinitely in a refrigerator, or stored in a frost-free frozen section of a refrigerator.

D. If the laboratory must save serum or plasma for testing later, it should be stored in a freezer at or below −20 degrees C. It should also be kept covered. (pp. 195–196)

25.

A, B, D. Glycolytic action does *not* refer to lysing of the red blood cells or the white blood cells or to platelet activation.

C. Glycolytic action refers to the breakdown of glucose, which can interfere with the analysis of various chemical constituents such as glucose, calcitonin, aldosterone, phosphorus, and enzymes. (p. 197)

26.

A. An airtight container and icy water decrease the loss of gases from the specimen. (p. 197)

B. Coagulation is not promoted by icy water or an airtight container, nor is it desired for a blood gas analysis.

C. The container and icy water help to ensure an accurate and reliable result due to a properly handled specimen but do not have an effect on the instrumentation phase of testing.

D. The container and icy water do not increase the oxygen content in the specimen.

27.

A, B, C. Specimens that may require chilling include those being tested for gastrin, ammonia, lactic acid, renin, catecholamine, parathyroid hormone, pyruvate, and blood gas analyses.

D. Specimens that may require chilling include those being tested for gastrin, ammonia, lactic acid, renin, catecholamine, parathyroid hormone, pyruvate, and blood gas analyses. Blood cultures do *not* need to be chilled. (pp. 197–198)

28.

A. Tepid water is lukewarm and will not keep the specimen cool.

B. A freezer unit may actually freeze the specimen, causing loss of its integrity and erroneous results.

C. Icy water or slushy water will keep the specimen cool and will not freeze it. (p. 197)

D. Frozen blocks of ice may freeze the specimen during transport.

29.

A. Specimens for CBC, diff, and platelet counts are not light-sensitive and do not need to be protected in a special manner.

B. Specimens for PT and PTTs are not light-sensitive and do not need to be protected in a special manner.

C. Bilirubin and some vitamins are light-sensitive and decompose if exposed to light. Specimens (blood or urine) being tested for these constituents should be protected from bright light with aluminum foil wrapping or other special containers designed to keep light out. (p. 199)

D. "None of the above" is not a correct answer.

30.

A. Specimens being tested for CBC, diff, and platelet counts do not require warming.

B. Specimens being tested for PT and PTTs do not require warming.

C. Specimens being tested for bilirubin and vitamins do not require warming.

D. Specimens that require warming to body temperature, 37°C, include those for testing cold agglutinins and cryofibrinogen. These special cases require a heat block or other appropriate warming device for transportation and handling purposes. (p. 199)

31.

A. Most laboratories require that primary specimen tubes be placed in a leakproof bag, not a biohazard box, to contain the specimen in case of breakage during transportation.

B. Most laboratories require that primary specimen tubes be placed in a leakproof bag to contain the specimen in case of breakage during transportation. (p. 196)

C and D. Neither aluminum foil nor icy water would contain a spoilage in case a specimen were to break during transportation.

32.

A. Blood and urine specimens for microbiological culture should be transported to the laboratory quickly so that the samples can be transferred to culture media, thereby enhancing the possibility of isolating pathogenic bacteria. Under normal circumstances, the blood cells will not rupture.

B. Blood and urine specimens for microbiological culture should be transported to the laboratory quickly to improve the likelihood of detecting pathogens. (p. 199)

C. Quick transportation to the laboratory is not likely to keep the specimens close to body temperature.

D. Under normal circumstances, exposure to light should not affect microbiological specimens.

33.

A. Hand-carrying the specimen is not the most efficient or safe way to transport specimens, even though it is commonly used.

B. Clear biohazard carts are not normally used.

C. The most efficient and safe method of specimen transportation in a large health care organization is through pneumatic tube systems. (pp. 199–200)

D. Email for specimens does not exist.

34.

A. Results should not be released immediately upon completion of the testing process.

B. The JCAHO and CAP state that laboratory results should be confirmed, dated, and a copy sent to the clinical record. (p. 202)

C. Calling the results to a physician is important if it was a "stat" request.

D. Faxing the results immediately to the patient is never appropriate without prior approval and documentation.

35.

A. Specimens such as human or animal feces; blood and blood components; body fluids such as spinal fluid, pleural fluid, or sputum; or biopsy tissues may need to be transported to reference or research laboratories. However, crime scene artifacts are not typically handled in a hospital clinical laboratory. (pp. 201–202)

B, C, D. Specimens such as human or animal feces; blood and blood components; body fluids such as spinal fluid, pleural fluid, or sputum; or biopsy tissues may need to be transported to reference or research laboratories. In packing or receiving one of these specimens, a special transport container must be used, with special attention to preventing leakage, temperature and pressure changes during transport, mislabeling, and breakage.

36.

A, B, C. CAP recommends that in designing a laboratory report form, the following issues should be considered: identification of patient and physician, patient location, date and time of specimen collection, source and description of specimen, precautions, packaging requirements for the specimen, understandability of the report, ability to be located in the patient's clinical record, reference ranges, and abnormal values.

D. CAP recommends that in designing a laboratory report form, the following issues should be considered: identification of patient and physician, patient location, date and time of specimen collection, source and description of specimen, precautions, packaging requirements for the specimen, understandability of the report, ability to be located in the patient's clinical record, reference ranges, and abnormal values. Patient and physician addresses are *not* required. (p. 202)

37.

A. A blood drawing list, or log sheet, can serve to provide a record of specimens that have been collected throughout the day. For hospital use, a copy could be located on a nursing unit as well as in the laboratory. (p. 193)

B. The log book/sheet would not serve to keep information confidential.

C. The log book/sheet would not serve to keep track of employee productivity.

D. The log book/sheet would not serve to track quality control of supplies/reagents.

38.

A, B, C. Pneumatic tube systems can be used to transport patient records, messages, letters, bills, medications, X-rays, and laboratory specimens. In considering the system for specimen transport, the following factors are important to maintain specimen integrity: mechanical reliability, distance of transport, speed of carrier, landing mechanism, effect on the chemical and cellular components of specimens, sizes of the carriers, shock absorbency, and radius of the loops and bends in the system.

D. Pneumatic tube systems can be used to transport patient records, messages, letters, bills, medications, X-rays, and laboratory specimens. In considering the system for specimen transport, the following factors are important to maintain specimen integrity: mechanical reliability, distance of transport, speed of carrier, landing mechanism, effect on the chemical and cellular components of specimens, sizes of the carriers, shock absorbency, and radius of the loops and bends in the system. Quality control of supplies would *not* have a direct effect on its use. (pp. 199–200)

39.

A. Handwritten labels are more prone to transcription errors.

B. Computerized labels using bar codes provide the most accurate and efficient labels that can be generated. (p. 189)

C. An addressograph machine can also be used to make labels and is generally very reliable; however, it is not as efficient or reliable as computerized barcoded labels.

D. The use of prelabeled specimen tubes is not recommended.

40.

A. Quality-control information usually contains facts about the following: hazards associated with the use of a reagent or supplies, proper use and storage information, expiration dates and stability information, and indications for measuring the precision and accuracy of the analytical process to be involved. Employee health information is *not* normally included in QC data. (p. 186)

B, C, D. Quality-control information usually contains facts about the following: hazards associated with the use of a reagent or supplies, proper use and storage information, expiration dates and stability information, and indications for measuring the precision and accuracy of the analytical process to be involved.

41.

A. Bar codes have not been used to determine the patient's arm preferences. However, they have many applications in specimen identification, processing, and testing, including patient names, date of birth (DOB), identification numbers, test codes, accession numbers, billing codes, product numbers, and inventory records. (p. 191)

B, C, D. Bar codes have many applications in specimen identification, processing, and testing, including patient names, date of birth (DOB), identification numbers, test codes, accession numbers, billing codes, product numbers, and inventory records.

42.

A. Transportation variables that affect the preanalytical phases of specimen handling include specimen leakage, specimen tube breakage in the pneumatic tube, and excessive shaking in the transport vehicle. (pp. 184–85)

B. Inadequate centrifugation is considered a processing error.

C. Inadequate volume in the test tube is considered a preventable specimen variable or error that may be controlled by the phlebotomist.

D. Patient stress and anxiety are also preanalytical variables that may affect the process but are not related to the transportation of the specimen.

43.

A. Tube breakage is usually due to transportation or processing error.

B. Inadequate centrifugation is considered a processing error.

C. Inadequate volume in the test tube is controlled by the phlebotomist.

D. Patient variables that affect the preanalytical process are stress and anxiety, diurnal variations, refusal to cooperate, fasting condition, and availability. (pp. 184–185)

44.

A, B, C. Processing variables that affect the preanalytical process include inadequate centrifugation, delays in processing, contamination of the specimen, exposure to heat or light, and excessive shaking or mixing.

D. Processing variables that affect the pre-analytical process include inadequate centrifugation, delays in processing, contamination of the specimen, exposure to heat or light, and excessive shaking or mixing. However, instrumentation malfunctions usually occur during the "analytical" phase of testing. (pp. 184–185)

45.

A. Another name for a "critical value" is "panic value," *not* "radical value."

B. Another name for a "critical value" is "panic value," *not* "random value."

C. Another name for a "critical value" is "panic value." (p. 203)

D. Another name for a "critical value" is "panic value," *not* "static value."

46.

A and B. The caller should be greeted and acknowledged and asked whether he or she may be placed on hold. If the caller has an emergency, this gives him or her an opportunity to state it. If the caller is immediately placed on hold, the urgency or nature of the call remains unknown.

C. Mary should have stopped her work temporarily to answer the phone or asked for assistance. If she had no assistance, she should have greeted the caller in a polite and professional manner, stated the department name, and asked how she could help. She should have restated the request or asked for clarification and documented it. (p. 187)

D. This statement did not allow the caller to speak and is not appropriate.

47.

A, C, D. The telephone is the most frequently used method of live communication in any setting. It is vitally important that health care workers be aware of the procedures for operating it and the etiquette for professional dialogue. Training can include effective customer service manners, transferring calls, placing someone on hold, using an intercom system, using voice mail, organizing conference calls, using speakerphones, documenting complete messages, and appropriate greetings.

B. In this case, Mary seems to have a working knowledge of the processing techniques that most likely include centrifugation. Therefore, this would be a lower priority for her continued education. The focus of her training should be those mentioned above. (p. 187)

48.

A. Many types of technology are available to enhance effective communication; however, a satellite radio would probably not improve the situation. (p. 187)

B, C, D. Many types of technology are available to enhance effective communication. Each facility needs to evaluate the cost and reliability of various products; however, among the communication devices that are commonly used in the specimen processing and collection areas are fax machines, speakerphones, voice mail, intercom systems, telephone headsets, bar code printers and scanners, and various types of computers.

49–50.

A through D. (Correct answers are C and D, respectively.) There are serious fines and legal implications if employers and employees do not comply with the procedures for shipping specimens that are potentially biohazardous. The employers' responsibilities include providing information and training to employees who will be handling these specimens, assuring that specimens are properly identified, classified, packed, labeled, and documented accordingly, making arrangements with the mail carriers on all shipping details, and confirming delivery. It is the employees' responsibility to comply with all the above policies. (It is *not* the employers' nor employees' responsibility to provide security through customs.) In this case scenario, it appears that the technician might not have been completely trained, or she had forgotten the procedures, and/or could not find the appropriate procedure. General packing requirements involve a primary watertight package and secondary package with absorbent material in between the containers. Some specimens need to be chilled or frozen, thus requiring a refrigerant or dry ice. With increased attention to security and biohazardous risks, it is imperative that individuals be competent about transporting blood specimens. (pp. 200–201)

8 Blood Collection Equipment

chapter objectives

Upon completion of Chapter 8, the learner is responsible for the following:

➤ List the various types of anticoagulants used in blood collection, their mechanisms for preventing blood from clotting, and the vacuum collection tube color codes for these anticoagulants.

➤ Describe the latest phlebotomy safety supplies and equipment, and evaluate their effectiveness in blood collection.

➤ Identify the various supplies that should be carried on a specimen collection tray when a skin puncture specimen must be collected.

➤ Identify the types of equipment needed to collect blood by venipuncture.

➤ Describe the special precautions that should be taken and the techniques that should be used when various types of specimens must be transported to the clinical laboratory.

DIRECTIONS Each of the questions or incomplete statements below is followed by four suggested answers or completions. Select one answer that is best in each case.

1. Figure 8.1 can be used to collect specimens for:
   A. arterial blood gas measurement
   B. blood cultures
   C. microhematocrit measurement
   D. venous glucose testing

2. Cytogenetic analysis requires whole blood collected in a:
   A. green-topped tube
   B. red-topped tube
   C. gray-topped tube
   D. light blue–topped tube

3. The vials shown in Figure 8.2 are used in the collection of:
   A. microscopy specimens
   B. clinical chemistry specimens
   C. clinical immunology specimens
   D. microbiology specimens

4. Lithium heparin is a suitable anticoagulant for which of the following studies?
   A. erythrocyte sedimentation rate
   B. zinc level
   C. glucose level
   D. lithium level

5. Which of the following anticoagulants is found in a royal blue–topped blood collection tube?
   A. lithium heparin
   B. no anticoagulant
   C. sodium citrate
   D. ammonium heparin

6. The yellow-topped vacuum collection tube has which of the following additives?
   A. EDTA
   B. lithium heparin
   C. trisodium citrate
   D. sodium polyanetholesulfonate (SPS)

FIGURE 8.1.

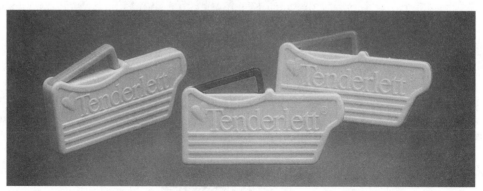

Courtesy of ITC, Edison, NJ.

FIGURE 8.2.

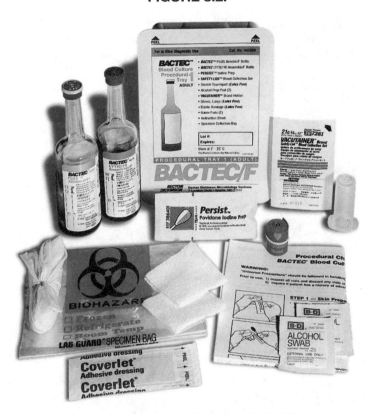

Courtesy of BD (Becton-Dickinson and Company), Sparks, MD.

7. What anticoagulant is preferred for the collection of whole blood in order to collect blood for STAT situations in clinical chemistry?

A. heparin

B. sodium citrate

C. EDTA

D. sodium oxalate

8. The blood collection set shown in Figure 8.3 is frequently used with the needle gauge size of:

A. 23

B. 19

C. 18

D. 17

9. For newborns, the penetration depth of lancets for blood collection must be less than:

A. 3.0 mm

B. 2.8 mm

C. 2.4 mm

D. 2.0 mm

10. The blood collection device shown in Figure 8.4 can be used for:

A. microcollection of blood for sed rate

B. ABO group and type blood collection

C. microcollection and dilution of blood samples for the WBC count

D. microcollection of blood for culture and sensitivity testing

FIGURE 8.3.

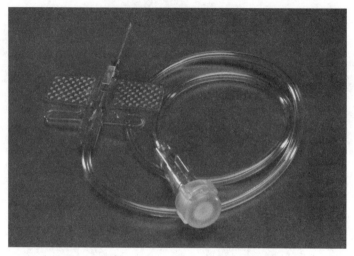

Courtesy of Tyco Healthcare/Kendall Co., LP, Mansfield, MA.

11. Which of the following additives prevent coagulation of blood by removing calcium through the formation of insoluble calcium salts?

A. ammonium oxalate, EDTA, sodium heparin

B. EDTA, lithium heparin, sodium citrate

C. sodium fluoride, lithium heparin, EDTA

D. EDTA, sodium citrate, potassium oxalate

12. Which of the listed needle gauges has the smallest diameter?

A. 19

B. 20

C. 21

D. 23

13. If the phlebotomist collects only venipuncture specimens, which of the following items would *not* be needed on his or her specimen collection tray?

A. disposable gloves

B. tourniquet

C. alcohol, iodine, and Betadine pads

D. Tenderletts (ITC, Edison, NJ)

14. A blood cell count requires whole blood collected in a:

A. green-topped tube

B. purple-topped tube

FIGURE 8.4.

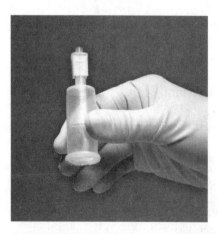

Courtesy of BD VACUTAINER Systems, *Preanalytical Solutions,* Franklin Lakes, NJ.

C. gray-topped tube

D. light blue–topped tube

15. The Monoject Monoletter (Tyco/Healthcare/Kendall, Mansfield, MA) is a:

A. safety device for collecting arterial blood gas specimens

B. safety device for collecting specimens by venipuncture

C. safe method to dispose of sharps

D. safety device for collecting capillary blood

16. Specimens for which of the following tests must be collected in light blue–topped blood collection tubes?

A. APTT

B. RPR test

C. VDRL

D. Selenium

17. Which of the following tests usually requires blood collected in a brown-topped blood collection vacuum tube?

A. cortisol level

B. CBC level

C. lactate dehydrogenase level

D. lead level

18. Which of the following is frequently used in the microcollection of electrolytes and general chemistry blood specimens?

A. BD Unopette

B. AVL Microsampler

C. Helena Pumpette

D. BD Microtainer

19. Which of the following is a commonly used intravenous device that is sometimes used in the collection of blood from patients who are difficult to collect blood by conventional methods?

A. Microvette capillary blood collection system

B. BD Unopette

C. butterfly needle

D. BD Microtainer

20. The glycolytic inhibitor is found in the:

A. green-topped tube

B. purple-topped tube

C. gray-topped tube

D. light blue–topped tube

21. Which of the following anticoagulants is found in a purple-topped blood collection vacuum tube?

A. EDTA

B. sodium heparin

C. ammonium oxalate

D. sodium oxalate

22. Alkaline phosphatase absolutely cannot be collected in which of the following tubes?

A. gray-topped tube

B. speckled-topped tube

C. red-topped tube

D. gold-topped tube

23. A prefilled device used as a collection and dilution unit is the:

A. BD Unopette

B. Vacuette tube

C. heparinized microcollection tube

D. Safe-T-Fill Capillary Blood Collection device

24. Which of the following devices was developed specifically for the bleeding time assay?
    A. Surgicutt
    B. Autolet Lite Clinisafe
    C. Tenderlett
    D. Unopette

25. The color coding for needles indicates the:
    A. length
    B. gauge
    C. manufacturer
    D. anticoagulant

26. Which of the following blood analytes is sensitive to light?
    A. lead
    B. glucose
    C. calcium
    D. bilirubin

27. Which of the following anticoagulants is used frequently in coagulation blood studies?
    A. citrate–phosphate–dextrose (CPD)
    B. potassium oxalate
    C. acid–citrate–dextrose (ACD)
    D. sodium citrate

28. Which of the following is a serum separation tube?
    A. heparinized microcollection tube
    B. microhematocrit tube
    C. winged infusion set
    D. SST tube

29. When blood is collected from a patient, the serum should be separated from the blood cells as quickly as possible to avoid:
    A. hemoconcentration
    B. hemolysis

C. glycolysis
D. hemostasis

30. Blood collected for creatine kinase *cannot* be collected in a:
    A. red-topped tube
    B. gray-topped tube
    C. speckled-topped tube
    D. gold-topped tube

31. Criteria used to describe vacuum collection tube size are:
    A. external tube diameter, maximum amount of specimen to be collected, and external tube length
    B. external tube diameter, minimum amount of specimen that can be collected, and external tube length
    C. internal tube diameter, maximum amount of specimen to be collected, and external tube length
    D. internal tube diameter, minimum amount of specimen that can be collected, and internal tube length

32. The evacuated tube system requires:
    A. a special plastic adapter, a syringe, and an evacuated sample tube
    B. an evacuated sample tube, a plastic adapter, and a double-pointed needle
    C. a double-pointed needle, a plastic holder, and a winged infusion set
    D. a special plastic adapter, an anticoagulant, and a double-pointed needle

33. The phlebotomist traveled to the home of 85-year-old Mrs. Ruth Harrison to collect blood for the PT, APTT, and potassium levels. Even though the blood collection was performed by using a winged infusion set on

Mrs. Harrison's fragile veins, the light blue–topped tube was underfilled. However, the required amount of blood was collected in the green-topped tube. Which of the following will most likely occur?

A. The potassium value will be falsely elevated.

B. The PT and PTT results will be falsely prolonged.

C. The potassium value will be falsely decreased.

D. The PT and PTT results will not be affected.

34. Blood for lead levels needs to be collected in a:

A. light blue–topped tube

B. purple-topped tube

C. tan-topped tube

D. green-topped tube

35. Measurement of blood copper, a trace element, requires blood collection in a:

A. light blue–topped tube

B. green-topped tube

C. royal blue–topped tube

D. purple-topped tube

36. Which of the following containers is frequently used for the micromeasurement of packed red cell volume?

A. BD Unopette

B. microhematocrit tube

C. BD Microtainer

D. S-Monovette Blood Collection System

37. The item in Figure 8.5 is usually referred to as a:

A. Samplette capillary blood collector

B. BD Microtainer

FIGURE 8.5.

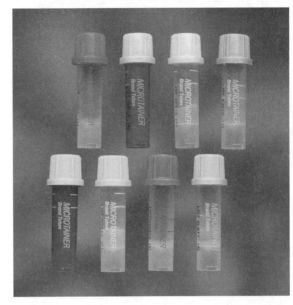

Source: See page 136.

C. Safe-T-Fill Capillary Blood Collection Device

D. BD Unopette

38. Which of the following anticoagulants is found in a green-topped blood collection vacuum tube?

A. EDTA

B. sodium heparin

C. sodium citrate

D. potassium oxalate

39. Which of the following anticoagulants allows preparation of blood films with minimal distortion of WBCs?

A. lithium heparin

B. sodium citrate

C. EDTA

D. sodium heparin

40. The anticoagulant lithium heparin is most appropriate for blood collection to perform:
    A. measurement of folate levels
    B. potassium
    C. measurement of lithium levels
    D. PT and APTT

41. Which of the following is an anticoagulant used in blood donations?
    A. sodium citrate
    B. acid citrate dextrose
    C. ethylene–diamine tetra–acetic acid
    D. lithium iodoacetate

42. Which of the following contains an antiglycolytic agent?
    A. light blue–topped tube
    B. purple-topped tube
    C. gray-topped tube
    D. green-topped tube

43. John, a phlebotomist who collects only capillary blood from patients in the newborn and pediatric units, probably would have all of the following equipment on his blood collection tray except:
    A. BD Unopettes
    B. sterile gauze pads
    C. serum separator BD VACUTAINER tubes
    D. biohazardous waste container for sharps

44. The maximum volume of blood that generally can be collected from a newborn (6 to 8 lbs.) during a hospital stay of 1 month or less is:
    A. 15 mL
    B. 23 mL
    C. 53 mL
    D. 60 mL

45. The red and black speckled-topped blood collection tube should be gently inverted five times so that blood clotting occurs in:
    A. 5 minutes
    B. 15 minutes
    C. 30 minutes
    D. 45 minutes

46. To avoid microclotting in the blood collection tube, it is extremely important that the blood collected in a purple-topped tube be gently inverted a minimum of:
    A. 0 times
    B. 5 times
    C. 8 times
    D. 12 times

47. The physician requested that a creatine kinase procedure be performed on Mrs. Billingsworth in Room 4220. The phlebotomist needs to collect the blood required for the procedure in a:
    A. red and black-topped tube
    B. light blue–topped tube
    C. gray-topped tube
    D. black-topped tube

48. The highest percentage of needlestick injuries has been shown to occur using the:
    A. 22-gauge needle with the evacuated tube system
    B. syringe needle
    C. S-Monovette
    D. winged infusion sets

49. ESR is the same laboratory assay as:
    A. estradiol
    B. erythrocyte sedimentation rate
    C. E-rosette receptor
    D. ethosuximide

50. Which of the following is the best for the sterile blood collection of trace elements, toxicology, and nutritional studies?

    A. gold-topped tube
    B. royal blue–topped tube
    C. purple-topped tube
    D. yellow-topped tube

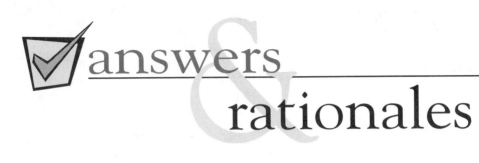

answers & rationales

1.

A, B, D. Figure 8.1 is the Tenderlett Automated Skin Incision Device (ITC, Edison, NJ) that is used to make a skin puncture in the finger or heel for the collection of capillary blood used for microhematocrit measurements and other clinical laboratory tests performed on capillary blood.

C. Figure 8.1 is the Tenderlett Automated Skin Incision Device (ITC, Edison, NJ) that is used to make a skin puncture in the finger or heel for the collection of capillary blood used for microhematocrit measurements and other clinical laboratory tests performed on capillary blood. (p. 232)

2.

A. Cytogenetic analysis requires whole blood collected in a green-topped (Na heparin) blood collection tube. (p. 213)

B. Red-topped tubes contain no additive, but sodium heparin is required for chromosome analysis.

C. Gray-topped tubes contain potassium oxalate and sodium fluoride or lithium iodoacetate and heparin, which will interfere in chromosome analysis.

D. Light blue–topped tubes contain sodium citrate, which will interfere in chromosome analysis.

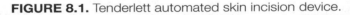

FIGURE 8.1. Tenderlett automated skin incision device.

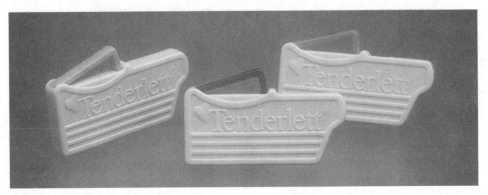

Courtesy of ITC, Edison, NJ.

3.

A. Microscopy specimens are usually urine collections and therefore do not require a blood collection system.

B. Clinical chemistry specimens do not require culture media vials, as shown in Figure 8.2.

C. Clinical immunology specimens do not require culture media vials, as shown in Figure 8.2.

D. The BD BACTEC culture vials shown in Figure 8.2 (courtesy of Becton-Dickinson and Company, Sparks, MD) are used for microbiology blood collections. (p. 214)

4.

A. The erythrocyte sedimentation rate requires a black-topped tube with sodium citrate or purple-topped tubes with EDTA.

B. Zinc levels may be erroneous if collected with lithium heparin, since the green-topped tubes are not manufactured for trace element collections.

C. Lithium heparin is found in green-topped tubes and is very suitable for blood glucose measurements. (p. 212)

D. The blood lithium level will be falsely increased if collected with lithium heparin anticoagulant.

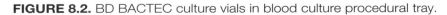

FIGURE 8.2. BD BACTEC culture vials in blood culture procedural tray.

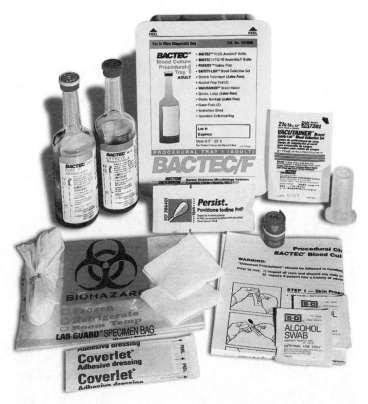

Courtesy of BD (Becton-Dickinson and Company), Sparks, MD.

5.

A. Lithium heparin is generally found in green-topped tubes, not royal blue.

B. Royal blue-topped tubes generally contain sodium heparin, EDTA, or no anticoagulant. (p. 211)

C. Sodium citrate is generally used in light blue–topped tubes.

D. Ammonium heparin is not generally used in blood collection tubes.

6.

A. EDTA is used in purple-topped collection tubes.

B. Lithium heparin is generally used in green-topped tubes.

C. Trisodium citrate is normally used in light blue–topped tubes.

D. Sodium polyanetholesulfonate (SPS) is used in the collection of blood culture specimens. (p. 214)

7.

A. Heparinized whole blood has become the specimen of choice for the clinical chemistry instruments used in STAT situations. (p. 209)

B. Sodium citrate is not the anticoagulant of choice for the clinical chemistry instruments used in STAT situations.

C. EDTA is not the anticoagulant of choice for the clinical chemistry instruments used in STAT situations.

D. Sodium oxalate is not the anticoagulant of choice for the clinical chemistry instruments used in STAT situations.

8.

A. The needle sizes of 21-, 23-, and 25-gauge are generally used with the blood collection set (courtesy of Tyco Healthcare/Kendall Co., LP, Mansfield, MA). (p. 221)

B. The needle size of 19-gauge is generally not used with a blood collection set, since it has a large interior bore.

C. The needle size of 18-gauge is generally not used with a blood collection set, since it has a large interior bore.

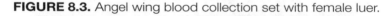

FIGURE 8.3. Angel wing blood collection set with female luer.

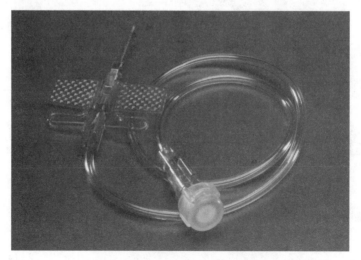

Courtesy of Tyco Healthcare/Kendall Co., LP, Mansfield, MA.

D. The needle size of 17-gauge is generally not used with a blood collection set, since it has a large interior bore.

9.

A. A depth of 3.0 mm can possibly penetrate bone in a newborn.

B. A depth of 2.8 mm can possibly penetrate bone in a newborn.

C. A depth of 2.4 mm can possibly penetrate bone in a newborn.

D. For newborns, lancets with tips less than 2.0 mm are required to avoid penetrating bone. (p. 230)

10.

A. The sed rate procedure requires undiluted whole blood, and therefore, the Unopette—a collection and dilution unit—cannot be used.

B. The ABO group and type blood collection procedure requires whole blood or serum, and therefore the diluting fluid in the Unopette cannot be used.

C. The Unopette shown in Figure 8.4 (courtesy of BD VACUTAINER Systems, Franklin Lakes, NJ) is a collection and dilution unit used for various procedures, including the WBC count, RBC count, platelet count, hemoglobin, RBC fragility, and sodium, potassium, and lead determinations. (p. 236)

D. Blood collection for blood cultures requires at least 3 mL of whole blood collected in culture vials or SPS tubes, not in a microcollection and dilution Unopette vial.

11.

A. Ammonium oxalate and EDTA prevent coagulation of blood by removing calcium and forming insoluble calcium salts. However, heparin prevents coagulation by inactivating blood-clotting thrombin and thromboplastin.

B. EDTA and sodium citrate prevent blood coagulation by removing calcium through the formation of insoluble calcium salts. However, lithium heparin prevents blood clotting by inactivating thrombin and thromboplastin.

C. Sodium fluoride is an additive to inhibit glycolytic action (glucose breakdown). Lithium heparin prevents coagulation by inactivating blood clotting thrombin and thromboplastin. EDTA does prevent blood coagulation through the formation of insoluble calcium salts.

D. Coagulation of blood can be prevented by the addition of oxalates, citrates, and/or EDTA by their ability to remove calcium, forming insoluble calcium salts. (p. 211)

12.

A, B, C. The smaller the gauge number, the larger the diameter of the needle.

D. The smaller the gauge number, the larger the diameter of the needle. (p. 220)

FIGURE 8.4. Unopette, a collection and dilution unit for blood samples.

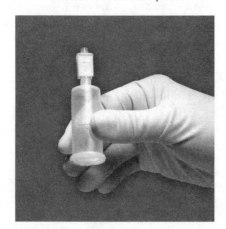

Courtesy of BD VACUTAINER Systems, *Preanalytical Solutions,* Franklin Lakes, NJ.

13.

A. Disposable gloves need to be worn for any kind of blood collection.

B. The tourniquet is needed to slow down venous flow for venipuncture.

C. Alcohol, iodine, and Betadine pads are cleansing agents that are needed in venipuncture to cleanse the blood collection site.

D. Tenderletts (ITC, Edison, NJ) are safe, single-use, automatically retracting, disposable devices used for microcollection by skin puncture. (pp. 231–232)

14.

A. Green-topped tubes contain heparin that can alter the accuracy of blood cell counts.

B. A blood cell count, including WBC count, RBC count, hemoglobin (Hgb), hematocrit (Hct), mean corpuscular volume (MCV), mean corpuscular hemoglobin (MCH), and mean corpuscular hemoglobin concentration (MCHC), requires whole blood collected in a purple-topped blood collection tube. (p. 213)

C. Gray-topped tubes contain sodium fluoride and potassium oxalate or lithium iodoacetate and heparin. These additives can falsely alter the blood cell count levels.

D. Light blue–topped tubes contain sodium citrate and will alter the accuracy of the blood cell count levels.

15.

A. The Monoject Monoletter is a safety device for skin puncture rather than arterial puncture.

B. The Monoject Monoletter is a safety device for skin puncture rather than venipuncture.

C. The Monoject Monoletter is a safety device for skin puncture with an enclosed lancet. Therefore, it is not for disposal of sharps.

D. The Monoject Monoletter is a safety device for skin puncture. (p. 231)

16.

A. The APTT (activated partial thromboplastin time) requires blood collection in the light blue–topped tubes containing citrate. (p. 213)

B. The RPR tests is a syphilis test requiring serum collected in red- or speckled-topped tubes.

C. The VDRL test is used to detect syphilis in blood and requires a red- or speckled-topped tube for collection.

D. Selenium (Se) is a trace element and must be tested on blood collected in a trace element tube (royal blue–topped with heparin) or in EDTA (purple-topped tube).

17.

A. Cortisol is a hormone, and to measure it, blood needs to be collected in a green-topped tube.

B. CBC level requires blood collected in EDTA—a purple-topped tube.

C. The enzyme, lactate dehydrogenase, needs to be detected in a blood sample collected with a speckled-topped tube.

D. Lead levels in blood are very minute and require a blood collection tube without any detectable lead such as the brown-topped tube. (p. 213)

18.

A. The BD Unopette can be used for blood measurements of sodium and potassium. However, this device is not used for general chemistry blood sampling.

B. The AVL microsampler is used for the collection of arterial blood required for blood gas analysis.

C. The Helena Pumpette is not a microcollection device.

D. The BD Microtainer tube is frequently used in the microcollection of electrolytes and general chemistry blood specimens. (p. 233)

19.

A. The Microvette capillary blood collection system is used to collect and store capillary blood specimens.

B. The BD Unopette is a microcollection and dilution device that is used to measure various analytes.

C. The butterfly needle, also referred to as a winged infusion set, is the most commonly used intravenous device. (p. 221)

D. The BD Microtainer is a microcollection device that is used to collect blood from a skin puncture site.

20.

A. The green-topped tube contains heparin, which is not a glycolytic inhibitor.

B. The purple-topped tube contains the anticoagulant EDTA and is not a glycolytic inhibitor.

C. The gray-topped tube contains a glycolytic inhibitor used in glucose testing. (p. 212)

D. The light blue–topped tube contains citrate, which is used as a glycolytic inhibitor.

21.

A. The anticoagulant EDTA is found in a purple-topped blood collection vacuum tube. (p. 213)

B. Sodium heparin is the anticoagulant used in green-topped blood collection vacuum tubes.

C. Ammonium oxalate is an anticoagulant that was used in the past but has been replaced by other additives.

D. Sodium oxalate is currently not used as an anticoagulant and is therefore not in the purple-topped vacuum tube.

22.

A. The gray-topped tube contains sodium fluoride that destroys alkaline phosphatase and many other enzymes in the blood. (p. 212)

B. The speckled-topped tube can be used for the collection of alkaline phosphatase.

C. The red-topped tube can be used for the collection of alkaline phosphatase.

D. The gold-topped tube cannot be used for the collection of alkaline phosphatase.

23.

A. The BD Unopette is a blood collection device that is prefilled with specific amounts of diluents or reagents. (pp. 233–234)

B. The Vacuette tube is a blood collection tube that does not have a diluent for dilution of the blood.

C. Heparinized microcollection tubes have an anticoagulant but are not prefilled with a solution for dilution of the blood.

D. The Safe-T-Fill Capillary Blood Collection device does not have solutions for dilution of the blood.

24.

A. Surgicutt is a sterile, standardized, disposable instrument that is used for bleeding time assay. (p. 226)

B. Surgicutt is a sterile, standardized, disposable instrument that is used for bleeding time assay.

C. The Tenderlett is a safety microcollection device.

D. The BD Unopette is a blood collection and dilution device used in the measurement of the RBC count, WBC count, platelet count, and other procedures but not bleeding time.

25.

A. The length of the needle is *not* indicated by a color code. The gauge of the needle is indicated by the color code.

B. The gauge size of the needle is identified by the color code on the sealed shield. (p. 220)

C. The color code on the shield indicates the gauge of the needle, not the manufacturer.

D. The blood collection tubes contain additives as shown by their tops. Needles have color-coded shields to indicate gauge size.

26.

A. Lead is an analyte that must be collected in a brown-topped vacuum tube, but it does not have to be protected from light.

B. Glucose is not chemically degraded when exposed to light, and therefore blood for glucose measurement does not require protection from light.

C. Calcium is not chemically degraded when exposed to light, and therefore blood collected for calcium determinations does not need to be protected from light.

D. Bilirubin breaks down chemically when exposed to light, and thus, the blood must be protected from light when bilirubin is to be measured. (p. 233)

27.

A. Citrate–phosphate–dextrose (CPD) is an anticoagulant and preservative that is frequently used in the collection of blood for blood donations.

B. Potassium oxalate is an anticoagulant that is used in the gray-topped vacuum tubes for blood glucose testing.

C. Acid–citrate–dextrose (ACD) is an anticoagulant and preservative that is frequently used in the collection of blood for blood donation.

D. Sodium citrate, the anticoagulant in light blue–topped blood collection tubes, is fre-

quently used in coagulation blood studies. (p. 213)

28.

A. The heparinized microcollection tube is a microcollection capillary tube that contains heparin to mix with the blood to avoid blood coagulation.

B. The microhematocrit tube is a microcollection capillary tube that contains heparin to mix with the blood to avoid blood coagulation.

C. The winged infusion set is a stainless steel beveled needle and tube with attached plastic wings.

D. The BD Vacutainer Serum Separator Tube (SST) (BD VACUTAINER Systems, Franklin Lakes, NJ) contains a separator barrier to separate the blood cells from the serum. (p. 215)

29.

A. Hemoconcentration sometimes occurs in the patient at the venipuncture site because of several factors, including prolonged tourniquet application, squeezing, and probing the site.

B. Hemolysis is the breakdown of RBCs, which is not the most critical reason for separating blood cells from the serum.

C. Glycolysis is the breakdown of glucose, which can lead to erroneously low blood glucose results if the red blood cells are not separated from the serum. (p. 212)

D. Hemostasis is the maintenance of circulating blood in the liquid state and retention of blood in the vascular system within the human body.

30.

A. Blood for creatine kinase can be collected in the red-topped tube, since it contains no interfering additives.

B. The gray-topped tube contains fluoride, which will break down the enzyme creatine kinase and give a falsely low level. (p. 212)

C. Blood for creatine kinase can be collected in the speckled-topped tube, since it separates serum from blood cells and has no effect on the creatine kinase level.

D. Blood for creatine kinase can be collected in the gold-topped tube, since it contains no interfering additives.

31.

A. The external tube diameter and length plus the maximum amount of specimen to be collected into the vacuum tube are the criteria that are used to describe vacuum collection tube size. (pp. 208–209)

B. Two criteria are correct: the external tube diameter and length. However, it is the maximum rather than minimum amount of specimen that can be collected as the third criterion.

C. Maximum amount of specimen to be collected and external tube length are two correct criteria. However, the third criterion is external rather than internal tube diameter.

D. All three criteria are incorrect for this distracter. The correct criteria should be external rather than internal tube diameter and tube length. Also, the third criterion should be the maximum rather than minimum amount of specimen to be collected.

32.

A. A syringe is not part of the evacuated tube system; the plastic adapter, evacuated sample tube, and double-pointed needle are the three parts of the system.

B. The evacuated tube system requires three components: the evacuated sample tube, the double-pointed needle, and a special plastic adapter. (p. 208)

C. The double-pointed needle and plastic holder are two parts of the evacuated tube system. However, the winged infusion set, also referred to as the butterfly, is not considered the third part of the evacuated tube system.

D. A special plastic adapter and double-pointed needle are two parts of the evacuated tube system; the third component is the evacuated sample tube rather than anticoagulant.

33.

A. The potassium value is determined from the blood collected in the green-topped tube. Since the required amount of blood was collected in this tube, the result should not be erroneously affected.

B. If a light blue–topped tube is underfilled, coagulation results will be erroneously prolonged. (p. 213)

C. The potassium value is determined from the blood collected in the green-topped tube. Since the required amount of blood was collected in this tube, the result should not be erroneously affected.

D. The PT and PTT tests are performed on blood collected with the anticoagulant sodium citrate. If the required blood level is not collected in the sodium citrate tube, then the ratio of sodium citrate to blood is increased, causing erroneously prolonged coagulation results.

34.

A. The light blue–topped tube is not the appropriate tube for collection of lead determinations.

B. The lead determinations should not be collected in a purple-topped tube.

C. The tan-topped tube has been designed for the collection of lead determinations. (p. 213)

D. The green-topped tube is not the appropriate tube for collection of lead determinations.

35.

A. The light blue–topped tube is not usually used for collection of blood for the blood copper procedure.

B. The green-topped tube contains the anticoagulant heparin and is usually used for chemistry tests, but not trace element testing.

C. The royal blue–topped tube is designed for collection of trace elements such as copper. (pp. 211, 213)

D. The purple-topped tube contains the anticoagulant EDTA and is generally used for hematology testing.

36.

A. The BD Unopette is a microcollection device that serves as a collection and dilution unit for the measurement of several analytes, including WBC count, RBC count, platelet count, and hemoglobin.

B. The microhematocrit tube contains heparin and is used for the collection of specimens to measure packed red blood cell volume. (p. 232)

C. The BD Microtainer is a microcollection tube that is used for blood collection to measure several chemistry analytes but not blood gas analysis.

D. The S-Monovette Blood Collection System is a multiple-sampling blood collection system for venipuncture collections, not microcollections.

37.

A. The Samplette capillary blood collection device (Tyco Healthcare/Kendall, Mansfield, MA) is not shown in Figure 8.5, but it is also a blood microcollection device.

B. The BD Microtainer (BD VACUTAINER Systems, Franklin Lakes, NJ) is shown in Figure 8.5 and is used frequently for electrolytes and general chemistry microspecimens. (pp. 233–234)

C. The Safe-T-Fill Capillary Blood Collection device (RAM Scientific Co., Needham, MA) is not

shown in Figure 8.5, but it is also used in the microcollection of blood for various analytes.

D. The BD Unopette (BD VACUTAINER Systems, Franklin Lakes, NJ) is not shown in Figure 8.5; it is a type of device that serves as a collection and dilution unit for blood samples.

38.

A. The anticoagulant EDTA is found in a purple-topped blood collection vacuum tube.

B. The anticoagulant sodium heparin is found in a green-topped blood collection vacuum tube. (p. 211)

C. The anticoagulant sodium citrate is found in a light blue–topped blood collection vacuum tube.

D. The anticoagulant potassium oxalate is found in a gray-topped blood collection vacuum tube.

39.

A. Lithium heparin is not suitable for blood smears because the anticoagulant interferes in the staining process.

FIGURE 8.5. BD Microtainer tube.

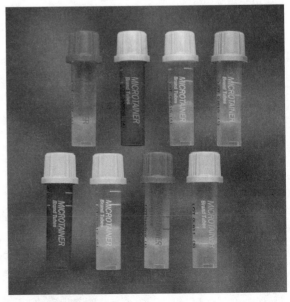

Courtesy of BD VACUTAINER Systems, *Preanalytical Solutions,* Franklin Lakes, NJ.

B. Sodium citrate is generally not used in the preparation of blood smears, since it can create alterations in the staining process.

C. Ethylene–diamine tetra–acetic acid (EDTA) is used to collect blood for blood smears, since it creates minimal distortion of WBCs. (p. 211)

D. Sodium heparin is not suitable for blood smears because the anticoagulant interferes in the staining process.

40.

A. The anticoagulant lithium heparin is not appropriate for blood collection to measure folate levels.

B. For potassium measurements, heparinized plasma or whole blood, rather than serum, is preferred. (p. 212)

C. The anticoagulant lithium heparin should not be used to collect blood for the measurement of lithium levels, since it will lead to a falsely elevated level.

D. PT and APTT are coagulation procedures that need blood collected with the anticoagulant sodium citrate.

41.

A. Sodium citrate is an anticoagulant that is generally used for collection of blood to test for coagulation abnormalities.

B. Acid citrate dextrose (ACD) is one of the anticoagulants that is used extensively in blood donations. (p. 210)

C. Ethylene–diamine tetra–acetic acid (EDTA) is the anticoagulant found in the purple-topped tube for hematology testing.

D. Lithium iodoacetate is the anticoagulant found in the gray-topped tube for glucose testing.

42.

A. The light blue–topped tube contains sodium citrate, which is an anticoagulant but not an antiglycolytic agent.

B. The purple-topped tube contains EDTA, which is an anticoagulant but not an antiglycolytic agent.

C. The gray-topped tube contains sodium fluoride or lithium iodoacetate, which are antiglycolytic agents. (p. 212)

D. The green-topped tube contains lithium or sodium heparin, which is an anticoagulant but not an antiglycolytic agent.

43.

A. Unopettes are blood collection and dilution devices used in microcollection for various assays.

B. Sterile gauze pads are required in both venipuncture and skin puncture.

C. Serum separator BD VACUTAINER tubes are used for venipuncture collections rather than microcollections. Since microcollection is the procedure used by the phlebotomist, he uses microcollection tubes rather than BD VACUTAINERS. (pp. 215, 230)

D. Biohazard waste containers for sharps are used for venipuncture and skin puncture procedures.

44.

A, C, D. The volume of cumulative blood to be collected during a hospital stay (1 month or less) from a newborn weighing 6 to 8 lbs is approximately 23 mL.

B. The volume of cumulative blood to be collected during a hospital stay (1 month or less) from a newborn weighing 6 to 8 lbs is approximately 23 mL. (p. 481, Appendix 5)

45.

A, B, D. The red and black speckled-topped blood collection tube should be gently inverted five times so that blood clotting occurs in 30 minutes.

C. The red and black speckled-topped blood collection tube should be gently inverted five times so that blood clotting occurs in 30 minutes. (in the back of the *Phlebotomy Handbook*)

46.

A, B, D. The purple-topped tube must be gently inverted at least eight times after blood collection to prevent clotting.

C. The purple-topped tube must be gently inverted at least eight times after blood collection to prevent clotting. (in the back of the *Phlebotomy Handbook*)

47.

A. Creatine kinase testing is a chemistry test and should occur in the red and black speckled-topped tube that yields blood cells and serum. (on back page of *Phlebotomy Handbook*)

B. Creatine kinase testing is a chemistry test and should occur from blood collected in a red and black speckled-topped tube. The light-blue topped tube is used mainly for coagulation testing.

C. Gray-topped tubes contain fluoride, which destroys the enzyme, creatine kinase.

D. Creatine kinase testing is a chemistry test and should occur in the red and black speckled-topped tube that yields blood cells and serum.

48.

A. The 22-gauge needle with an unguarded adapter needle apparatus can lead to needlestick injuries, but the winged-infusion sets account for the highest percentage of needlestick injuries.

B. The syringe with an unguarded needle can lead to needlestick injuries, but the winged-infusion sets account for the highest percentage of needlestick injuries.

C. The S-Monovette (Sarsedt, Inc., Newton, NC) is a safety device for vacuum collection or the syringe collection technique. It is designed to eliminate needlestick injuries.

D. Winged-infusion sets, also referred to as blood collection sets or the butterfly needle, have been shown to account for the highest percentage of needlestick injuries. (p. 222)

49.

A, C, D. ESR is the same laboratory assay as a sedimentation rate, erythrocyte sedimentation rate, or sed rate.

B. ESR is the same laboratory assay as a sedimentation rate, erythrocyte sedimentation rate, or sed rate. (p. 213)

50.

A. The gold-topped tube has a polymer barrier for the separation of clotted blood from serum and is used for general chemistry testing.

B. The royal blue–topped tube has been designed to collect sterile blood specimens for trace elements, toxicology, and/or nutritional studies. (p. 213)

C. The purple-topped tube contains the anticoagulant EDTA and is frequently used for hematology studies.

D. The yellow-topped tube contains sodium polyanetholesulfonate (SPS) for the collection of blood culture specimens.

9 Venipuncture Procedures

chapter objectives

Upon completion of Chapter 9, the learner is responsible for the following:

➤ Describe the patient identification process.

➤ List supplies used in a typical venipuncture procedure.

➤ Describe methods for hand hygiene.

➤ Identify the most common sites for venipuncture, and situations when these sites might not be acceptable. Identify alternative sites for the venipuncture procedure.

➤ Describe the process and the time limits for applying a tourniquet to a patient's arm.

➤ Describe the decontamination process and the agents that are used to decontaminate skin for routine blood tests and blood cultures.

➤ Describe the steps of a venipuncture procedure.

➤ Describe the "order of draw" for collection tubes.

➤ Explain the importance of collecting timed specimens at the requested times.

➤ Define the terms "fasting" and "STAT" when referring to blood tests.

DIRECTIONS Each of the questions or incomplete statements below is followed by four suggested answers or completions. Select one answer that is best in each case.

1. Which of the following steps is *not* usually part of each venipuncture procedure?
   A. hand hygiene
   B. patient identification and vein selection
   C. pulling long hair back into a ponytail
   D. selecting supplies and equipment

2. Prior to performing a venipuncture, why should a clean pair of gloves be put on in the presence of the patient?
   A. It is a federal law for all health care workers.
   B. It is a reassuring, safety-conscious gesture for both the patient and the worker.
   C. It saves time and money.
   D. It eliminates the need for repeated hand-hygiene techniques.

3. What is the importance of hand-hygiene techniques?
   A. It significantly reduces the number of outbreaks of infections.
   B. It prevents HBV infection after a needlestick.
   C. It helps with vein selection.
   D. It eliminates the use of gloves.

4. What does MRSA signify?
   A. Multiple Reasons for Safety Advice
   B. Methicillin Resistant Staphylococcus aureus
   C. Measures of Radiation Alert
   D. Mumps and Rubella Serum Antibodies

5. Identification of an inpatient can *best* be accomplished by which of the following?
   A. using the patient's hospital id bracelet and a verbal confirmation from the patient
   B. hospital room number and bed assignment
   C. confirmation from a patient's relative
   D. using the patient's hospital id bracelet and matching it with the test requisition

6. Information on an inpatient's identification bracelet always includes the:
   A. patient's name and identification number
   B. physician's name and laboratory tests usually ordered
   C. patient's bed assignment
   D. nearest relative and emergency phone number

7. If an inpatient has severe burns and does not have an identification bracelet, who should be asked to make the identification before a venipuncture?
   A. the patient's son or daughter
   B. another patient in the room
   C. the clerk who checked the patient in
   D. the nurse in charge of the patient

8. A requisition for laboratory tests, whether electronic or handwritten, must contain all of the following information *except:*
   A. patient's full name, identification number, and date of birth
   B. dates and types of tests to be performed

C. physician's name

D. social security number and password

9. Accidental needlestick injuries may lead to serious or fatal infections caused by which of the following:

A. anemia

B. HBV, HIV, HCV

C. leukemia

D. HIPAA

10. Hand lotions can be used in phlebotomy for which of the following purposes?

A. to finish the process of hand antisepsis

B. to maximize antiseptic action

C. to minimize the occurance of dermatitis

D. to provide lubrication prior to wearing gloves

11. What type of hand rub is usually acceptable for decontamination of hands prior to a venipuncture procedure?

A. saline-based

B. alcohol-based

C. rubs that are slightly acidic

D. lotion-based

12. How much hand rub is needed to decontaminate hands?

A. .5 mL

B. 1 mL

C. 5 mL

D. the amount that is recommended by the manufacturer

13. What is the best way to decontaminate a phlebotomist's hands if they are visibly dirty with dust and dirt?

A. Wash hands with soap and water.

B. Use an alcohol-based hand rub alone and wipe it off with paper towels.

C. Use antimicrobial wipes.

D. Wear sterile gloves.

14. Where is the anticubital area?

A. near the shoulder

B. at the biceps

C. slightly below the elbow

D. near the wrist

15. Identify the most common site for venipuncture.

A. median cubital vein

B. ulnar vein

C. basilic vein

D. radial vein

16. Select one reason for not using arm veins for a venipuncture.

A. The patient has IV lines or casts on both arms.

B. The patient is a child and is tempermental.

C. The patient is elderly and tends to fall asleep during the procedure.

D. The patient is frail and in pain.

17. If arm veins cannot be used for a venipuncture, the preferred alternative veins lie in the:

A. ankles or feet

B. anterior surface of the hand or wrist

C. dorsal side of the hand or wrist

D. outermost edge of the hand

18. Which of the following does *not* need to be included on the label of the blood specimen or body fluid specimen?

A. patient's name and identification number

B. the time that specimen is collected

C. the attending physician's name

D. social security number and password

19. What happens if the tourniquet pressure is too tight or prolonged on the arm prior to the venipuncture?
    A. Laboratory test results will likely be falsely elevated including cell counts and protein levels.
    B. Laboratory test results will not be affected.
    C. Only drug levels will be decreased.
    D. Tourniquet pressure will cause excessive bleeding after the procedure.

20. Where should the tourniquet be placed on the patient during the venipuncture procedure?
    A. slightly above the venipuncture site
    B. slightly underneath the venipuncture site
    C. about 3 inches above the venipuncture site
    D. at least 6 inches below the venipuncture site

21. Which of the following causes pooling of blood in veins?
    A. syringe method
    B. tourniquet
    C. capillary tube
    D. evacuated tube method

22. After a venipuncture site has been decontaminated with alcohol, which of the following is the appropriate step?
    A. Blow on the site to speed the drying process.
    B. Using the gloved hand, fan the site to assist in drying.
    C. Allow the site to air-dry.
    D. Continue immediately with the venipuncture.

23. Alcohol should be allowed to dry for how many seconds before the venipuncture?
    A. up to 5 seconds
    B. 6 to 10 seconds
    C. 11 to 15 seconds
    D. 30 to 60 seconds

24. During the venipuncture, what is the best angle for inserting the needle into the skin?
    A. 5–15 degrees
    B. 15–30 degrees
    C. 45–60 degrees
    D. 60–75 degrees

25. During the venipuncture procedure, after the needle is inserted and blood begins to flow, what should the phlebotomist do next?
    A. Release the tourniquet.
    B. Withdraw the needle.
    C. Release the adapter.
    D. Adjust the hub of the needle.

26. When the evacuated tube method is used for venipuncture, select the correct order of collection for the following tubes: blood culture tubes, coagulation tube, and hematology tube. Choose the order of tubes by their color of tube top.
    A. light blue, lavender, yellow blood culture tubes
    B. lavender, light blue, yellow blood culture tubes
    C. yellow blood culture tubes, light blue, lavender
    D. light blue, yellow blood culture tubes, lavender

27. Which of the following information is essential for labeling a patient's specimen?

A. the patient's name and identification number, date of collection, room number, and phlebotomist's initials

B. the patient's name and identification number, date of collection, time of collection

C. the patient's name and identification number, date and time of collection, phlebotomist's initials

D. the patient's name and identification number, date of collection, physician's name

28. The term "STAT" refers to:

A. abstaining from food over a period of time

B. using timed blood collections for specific specimens

C. using the early morning specimens for laboratory testing

D. immediate and urgent specimen collection

29. For which procedure(s) are povidone-iodine (Betadine) or iodine preparations used?

A. reduction of the pain of the needlestick

B. decontamination of the venipuncture site for all routine venipunctures

C. decontamination of the venipuncture site for blood culture specimens

D. coagulation testing only

30. Why is it important to get information about whether or not the patient has recently eaten?

A. Laboratory tests can be affected by the ingestion of food and drink.

B. Meals will likely make the patient vomit during the procedure.

C. After eating, patients usually have enlarged veins.

D. It is not that important to get this information.

31. How often should a health care worker's hands be decontaminated when duties require that many patients' venipunctures be performed during a short period of time?

A. after every two patients

B. after every five patients

C. at the beginning and end of a shift

D. before and after each patient

32. If a patient is obese, what special equipment would be helpful in the specimen collection process?

A. specially sized collection tubes

B. a face mask and gown

C. a large-sized blood pressure cuff and longer needle

D. a large-sized wheelchair and warming blankets

33. When a patient has "difficult" veins, which strategy would probably *not* improve the likelihood of a successful puncture?

A. slight rotation of the patient's arm to a different position

B. warming, then palpating the entire anticubital area to trace vein path

C. asking the patient for a preferred site

D. asking the doctor for a preferred site

34. Why is one side of the wrist more suitable for venipuncture than the other?

A. Nerves lie close to the palmar side and can easily be injured.

B. Veins are larger on the back side of the hand.

C. On the palmar side, one can more easily feel an artery.

D. all of the above

35. Arteries differ from veins in which of the following ways?
    A. thicker vessel walls with a pulsating feel
    B. more blue in color
    C. smaller in diameter
    D. the blood is warmer than in the veins

36. What venipuncture site should be considered first if a patient has had a mastectomy on the right side?
    A. the right arm
    B. the left arm
    C. the right hand
    D. the left hand

37. During a venipuncture procedure, the needle should always be inserted with the:
    A. bevel side down
    B. bevel side up
    C. bevel pointed away from the insertion site
    D. bevel perpendicular to the skin

38. What is a common concern if using the syringe method for venipuncture?
    A. excessive tissue fluid production
    B. cross-contamination of anticoagulants and needle safety
    C. the needle is too small
    D. it causes more pain

39. The winged infusion set is most useful for venipunctures in all but which *one* of the listed situations?
    A. young adult males
    B. small hand or wrist veins
    C. young children
    D. severely burned patients

40. After withdrawing a needle from a patient's arm, what step should be considered *immediately?*
    A. activating the safety device on the needle
    B. applying an adhesive bandage to the site
    C. labeling the specimen
    D. disposing of the needle

41. On occasion, specimens need to be rejected from laboratory testing. Which of the following factors may be used in this decision?
    A. The specimen is improperly transported.
    B. The specimen appears hemolyzed.
    C. The anticoagulated specimen contains blood clots.
    D. all of the above

42. In drawing blood for multiple laboratory tests some laboratories recommend that at least one other tube be drawn before the tubes for coagulation tests. What is the rationale behind this?
    A. To make sure that the coag tube is properly filled.
    B. To reduce the chances of contaminating the coag specimen with tissue fluids.
    C. To draw in the order that the tests will be performed in the laboratory.
    D. To ensure that the needle does not fall out.

43. When collecting blood in an evacuated tube with an anticoagulant, what is the importance of having the right volume of blood?
    A. It is important to maintaining homeostasis.
    B. It prevents hemolysis.
    C. It promotes bleeding.
    D. It provides the correct blood–additive ratio.

44. How should the anticoagulant be mixed with a blood specimen in an evacuated tube?
    A. Forcefully shaking the tube for 30 seconds.
    B. Centrifugation for 15 minutes.
    C. Mixing occurs naturally as the specimen is transported.
    D. Gentle inversion of the specimen.

45. The most commonly requested timed specimen is:
    A. glucose level
    B. cholesterol level
    C. triglycerides
    D. hemoglobin

46. Peak and trough levels are useful for what type of analyses?
    A. hormone levels
    B. therapeutic drug levels
    C. glucose screening
    D. gastric analysis

47. The term "butterfly" refers to the:
    A. safety device on a needle
    B. evacuated collection tube
    C. winged infusion set
    D. a syringe

48. In a routine situation, how can a phlebotomist minimize cross-contamination of anticoagulants and/or additives from one tube to the next during a multiple-sample venipuncture procedure?
    A. Keep the tube horizontal or slightly downward while filling.
    B. Treat the tubes as if they are hazardous.
    C. Always use a syringe to transfer blood to each tube.
    D. Draw the coagulation tube first.

Use the following scenario to refer to when answering Questions 49–51:

A health care worker entered a patient's room to draw blood specimens for the following tests: hematology cell counts, coagulation tests, blood cultures, and chemistry assays. The patient was an oncology patient and had scarring on many of her veins, had IVs in both forearms, and was a diabetic. Laboratory notes indicated that blood should not be drawn from this patient's feet. Answer the following questions about this scenario.

49. Which site would be most suitable for blood collection?
    A. earlobe
    B. heel of the foot
    C. posterior side of the hand or wrist
    D. the anterior surface of the wrist

50. What would be the preferred order of tube collection for these tests?
    A. blood cultures, coagulation, hematology, and chemistry
    B. blood cultures, chemistry, hematology, and coagulation
    C. hematology, coagulation, chemistry, and blood cultures
    D. coagulation, blood cultures, hematology, and coagulation

51. What measure could be taken to diminish the likelihood of complications when collecting blood for glucose, electrolytes, CBC, and PT?
    A. Use a butterfly system.
    B. Use a finger puncture.
    C. Decline to perform the venipuncture.
    D. Use a blood pressure cuff and tighten it more than usual to enhance pooling of the blood.

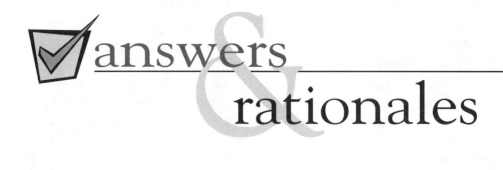

answers & rationales

1.

A,B,D. Hand hygiene, approaching, identifying, positioning the patient, and selecting supplies and equipment are included in the basic steps for every venipuncture.

C. Hand hygiene, approaching, identifying, positioning the patient, and selecting supplies and equipment are included in the basic steps for every venipuncture. However, combing and styling hair should be done prior to reporting to work and is not a part of a basic venipuncture procedure. (p. 246)

2.

A. It is *not* a federal law that health care workers wear gloves; however, it is recommended by federal and accrediting agencies for protective purposes.

B. Donning (putting-on) a clean pair of gloves in the presence of the patient provides a reassuring and safety-conscious gesture for the patient and the health care worker. (p. 247)

C. Donning gloves does not necessarily save time or money, but it is a safety-conscious practice.

D. Donning gloves does not eliminate the need to practice appropriate hand-hygiene techniques.

3.

A. Normal skin is colonized with microorganisms; therefore, the transmission of pathogens by health care workers can occur easily. Adherence to hand hygiene techniques (handwashing or use of alcohol-based hand rubs) has been shown to significantly reduce outbreaks of infections, including antimicrobial-resistant infections. (p. 247)

B. Hand-hygiene techniques cannot prevent an HBV infection after a needlestick.

C. Hand-hygiene techniques do not help with vein selection.

D. Hand-hygiene techniques do not eliminate the use of gloves. Rather, it is an extra measure of protection to prevent the transmission of infections.

4.

A. MRSA does not signify Multiple Reasons for Safety Advice.

B. MRSA signifies Methicillin-Resistant Staphylococcus aureus. (p. 247)

C. MRSA does not signify Measures of Radiation Alert.

D. MRSA does not signify Mumps and Rubella Serum Antibodies.

5.

A. Identification of an inpatient can *best* be accomplished by matching the patient's hospital identification bracelet with the test requisition. A verbal confirmation is also helpful but may be erroneous if the patient is sedated or has other types of mental impairment.

B. Hospital room number and bed assignment should not be used to identify a patient. Since room numbers and bed assignments are the last to be changed or replaced when patients are discharged or admitted to the hospital, they are less reliable as identifiers.

C. Confirmation from a patient's relative is helpful but should not be used as the only identifier for hospital inpatients.

D. Using the patient's hospital identification bracelet and matching it with the test requisition is the safest and most reliable way to confirm a patient's identity. Verbal confirmation is useful to reaffirm the identification, but not as a sole method. (p. 253)

6.

A. In addition to the patient's first and last names and identification number, the hospital identification bracelet may also include the patient's room number, bed assignment, and physician's name. (p. 252)

B,C,D. In addition to the patient's first and last names and identification number, the hospital identification bracelet may also include the patient's room number, bed assignment, and physician's name.

7.

A. A patient's child should not provide sole identity for the patient.

B. Another patient in the room should not identify the patient who is to have a venipuncture.

C. Clerical personnel are not usually responsible for making positive identifications for hospitalized patients unless authorized/confirmed by a nurse in charge.

D. If a hospitalized patient with severe burns does not have an identification bracelet, the nurse in charge of the patient should be asked to make the positive identification. This should be well documented. (p. 254)

8.

A,B,C. Laboratory requisitions for clinical testing, whether electronic or handwritten, must contain the patient's full name, identification number, and date of birth; the dates and types of tests to be performed; the physician's name, the location of the patient, and timing instructions.

D. Laboratory requisitions for clinical testing, whether computerized or handwritten, must contain the patient's full name, identification number, and date of birth; the dates and types of tests to be performed; the physician's name, the location of the patient, and timing instructions. (p. 250)

9.

A. Anemia cannot be caused by an accidental needlestick.

B. Accidental needlesticks are hazardous and can transmit bloodborne pathogens such as hepatitis B and C (HBV and HCV), and human immunodeficiency virus (HIV). (p. 247)

C. Leukemia is not transmitted by an accidental needlestick.

D. HIPAA is a federal regulation and not related to blood.

10.

A. Hand lotions do not provide antiseptic conditions.

B. Hand lotions do not maximize antiseptic action.

C. Hand lotions are used to relieve dryness caused by excessive hand-washing or excessive use of hand rubs. They minimize the occurrence of dermatitis associated with hand decontamination. (p. 248)

D. Hand rubs do not function to lubricate hands prior to wearing gloves. On the contrary, hands should be dry prior to donning gloves.

11.

A. Hand rubs for decontamination purposes are not referred to as "saline-based."

B. Alcohol-based hand rubs are effective for hand decontamination purposes if the hands are not visibly soiled. (p. 248)

C. Hand rubs for decontamination purposes are not referred to as "slightly acidic."

D. Lotion-based hand rubs are usually only for relieving dryness and are not suitable for decontamination purposes.

12.

A.–D. (The correct answer is D.) Phlebotomists should follow the manufacturer's recommended amount of hand rub to decontaminate hands. Usually it is a small amount that should be applied on one palm, then, while rubbing hands together, all surfaces of hands and fingers should be covered and rubbed until hands are dry. (p. 248)

13.

A. If hands are visibly dirty, contaminated, or soiled, they should be washed with either an

antimicrobial soap and water or a non-antimicrobial soap and water. (p. 248)

B. Alcohol based hand rubs are not as effective in removing dirty or soiled hands.

C. Antimicrobial wipes are not recommended for thorough removal of dirt from hands.

D. Hands should always be decontaminated before and after wearing gloves.

14.

A.–D. (The correct answer is C.) The anticubital area of the arm is just below the bend of the elbow. This is the most common site for venipuncture procedures.

15.

A. The most common site for venipuncture is in the antecubital area of the arm, in the median cubital vein. This vein lying close to the surface of the skin, is reportedly less painful. (p. 262)

B. The ulnar vein is not the most common site for venipuncture.

C. The basilic vein is also a commonly used vein for venipuncture and is also located in the antecubital area of the arm. However, it is not the most commonly used.

D. The radial vein is not the most common site for venipuncture.

16.

A. If a patient has an intravenous (IV) line or casts on both arms, the arms should not be used for performing a venipuncture. If the IV line or cast is only on one arm, the other arm may be used for venipuncture. (p. 267)

B. If the patient is a child, a venipuncture can still be performed by using appropriate pediatric methodologies.

C. If the patient is elderly, a venipuncture can be performed by using appropriate communication strategies and accommodations for the situation.

D. If the patient is frail, a venipuncture can be performed by using appropriate strategies to maximize the chances of a successful venipuncture and make the patient as comfortable as possible.

17.

A. Ankle or foot veins should only be used if arm veins and hand or wrist veins on the dorsal side are inaccessible. Most hospitals have special guidelines regarding phlebotomy procedures from the foot area because coagulation and vascular complications tend to be more troublesome in the lower extremities, especially for diabetic patients.

B. The anterior surface of the wrist has many nerves that can be damaged during venipuncture, and the procedure would be much more painful than other sites. It is not an acceptable site for venipuncture.

C. When arm veins cannot be used for venipuncture, the preferred site is the back of the hand or wrist, that is, the dorsal surface, *not* the palm side of the hand. (p. 268)

D. The outermost edge of the hand is not an appropriate site for venipuncture.

18.

A, B, C. Specimens should be labeled immediately at the patient's bedside or ambulatory setting, and the labels should contain the patient's full name and identification number, the date and time of collection, and the health care worker's initials. Other information that is helpful but optional is the patient's room number, bed assignment, or outpatient status.

D. Specimen labels do not need the patient's social security number and password. (p. 279)

19.

A. If a tourniquet is left on for more than 1 minute, it becomes uncomfortable and may cause blood to become hemoconcentrated. This could affect numerous laboratory tests, causing results to be elevated. Among the tests that may be affected are cell counts, coagulation factors, and protein levels. (p. 269)

B. If a tourniquet is left on for more than 1 minute, it becomes uncomfortable and may cause blood to become hemoconcentrated. This could affect numerous laboratory tests, causing results to be elevated. Among the tests that may be affected are cell counts, coagulation factors, and protein levels.

C. Prolonged tourniquet application would not decrease drug levels.

D. If a tourniquet is left on for more than 1 minute prior to venipuncture and removed at the appropriate time during the procedure, it is uncomfortable and not advisable but it should not cause excessive bleeding.

20.

A. The tourniquet should not be just slightly over the venipuncture site because it might get in the way during the procedure.

B. The tourniquet should not be underneath the venipuncture site because it would serve no useful purpose in that location.

C. A tourniquet should be applied about 3 inches above the venipuncture site. It should be tight but not painful and should be partially looped to allow for easy release with one hand. (p. 270)

D. The tourniquet should not be 6 inches below the venipuncture site because it would serve no useful purpose in that location.

21.

A. The syringe method does not cause pooling of blood in the veins.

B. A tourniquet causes pooling or filling of blood in veins. Such pooling makes blood collection easier during a venipuncture procedure, regardless of the method used to withdraw blood from the vein. (p. 269)

C. A capillary tube does not cause pooling of blood in the veins.

D. The evacuated tube method does not cause pooling of blood in the veins.

22.

A. Blowing on the site to speed the drying process may recontaminate the site.

B. Using a gloved hand to fan the site is not an appropriate action.

C. Alcohol should be allowed to air-dry for 30–60 seconds; this prevents recontamination, prevents stinging, and prevents the chances of contaminating the specimen with the alcohol. (p. 271)

D. The venipuncture should be continued only when the alcohol has been allowed to dry or it has been wiped off with sterile gauze.

23.

A. The alcohol will not dry in 5 seconds or less.

B. The alcohol will not dry in 6 to 10 seconds.

C. The alcohol will not dry in 10 to 15 seconds.

D. Alcohol should be allowed to air-dry for 30–60 seconds; this prevents recontamination, prevents stinging, and prevents the chances of contaminating the specimen with the alcohol. (p. 271)

24.

A. A 5- to 15-degree angle is not adequate to reach the vein and penetrate the skin properly.

B. The needle should be inserted in the same direction as the vein at a 15- to 30-degree angle to the skin. (p. 273)

C. A 45- to 60-degree angle might cause the needle to go too deeply into the arm.

D. A 60- to 75-degree angle also might cause the needle to go too deeply into the arm.

25.

A. After the needle is inserted and blood begins to flow, the tourniquet should be released, and the patient may open his or her fist. (p. 273)

B. The needle should not be withdrawn until all blood specimens have been collected in the appropriate tubes.

C. Releasing the adaptor is not an appropriate action.

D. Adjusting the hub of the needle is not usually necessary unless it was not properly attached before venipuncture.

26.

A, B, D. Blood culture tubes should always be drawn first, in this case followed by coagulation tubes and then hematology tubes.

C. Blood culture tubes (yellow-topped) are always collected first to reduce the chances of contamination. The coagulation tube (light blue-topped) should then be collected before the hematology tube (lavender-topped). (p. 277)

27.

A. The patient's room number, bed assignment, physician, or outpatient status is optional but useful information.

B. This information is incomplete; it is missing the phlebotomist's initials.

C. All specimen labels should include the patient's name and identification number, the date and time of collection, and the phlebotomist's initials. The patient's room number, bed assignment, or outpatient status is optional but useful information. (p. 279)

D. This information is incomplete; it is missing the time of collection and the phlebotomist's initials. The physician's name is useful but not required on a specimen label.

28.

A. Abstaining from food over a period of time is fasting.

B. Using timed blood collections is important for certain types of laboratory tests but does not refer to the term "STAT."

C. Using early-morning specimens is typical for most hospital laboratories and is usually a routine procedure, not a "STAT" situation.

D. The term "STAT" refers to an immediate or emergency condition. It indicates that a patient has a medical condition that is critical or likely to become critical. STAT blood collections should be drawn and analyzed immediately. (p. 284)

29.

A. Iodine does not reduce the pain of a needlestick.

B. Iodine may be used for the decontamination step of a venipuncture site for any routine venipunctures; however, more patients are allergic to it than to isopropanol, it takes more time to use, and it is not cost-effective.

C. Povidone-iodine preparations are used primarily for decontaminating the skin before venipuncture for blood gas analysis and blood cultures. Excess iodine should be removed from the skin with sterile gauze before the puncture. (p. 269)

D. "Coagulation testing only" is an inaccurate answer.

30.

A. Many laboratory tests can be affected by the ingestion of food and drink. It is important to note whether or not the patient has been fasting. (pp. 257–259)

B. Meals will not necessarily make a patient vomit during a venipuncture.

C. Eating does not cause patients to have enlarged veins.

D. It *is* very important to get this information.

31.

A, B, C. Hand decontamination only after every two or five patients or only at the beginning of a workshift could result in transmission of infections and is not an acceptable practice.

D. Hands should be decontaminated before and after each patient's specimen collection procedure. (pp. 247–248)

32.

A. Collection tubes should be the same ones used for other routine testing.

B. A mask or gown would not facilitate the venipuncture procedure.

C. Obese patients may require special equipment to facilitate the venipuncture procedure. This might include a large-sized blood pressure cuff to be used as a tourniquet and/or a longer needle for deeper penetration through the fatty layers to the vein. (p. 257)

D. A large-sized wheelchair would not facilitate the actual venipuncture procedure.

33.

A, B, C. To increase the likelihood of a successful puncture, several tips may help. These include slight rotation of the patient's arm to a different position, palpating the entire anticubital area to trace vein path, warming the site, gentle massaging, lowering the arm over the bedside, asking the patient for a preferred site, or using the other arm.

D. To increase the likelihood of a successful puncture, several tips may help. These include slight rotation of the patient's arm to a different position, palpating the entire anticubital area to trace vein path, warming the site, gentle massaging, lowering the arm over the bedside, asking the patient for a preferred site, or using the other arm. However, most doctors are not familiar with individual patients' veins so it is probably advisable *not* to ask the doctor about a preferred site unless unusual circumstances or complications arise. (pp. 262–267)

34.

A.–D. (The correct answer is D.) For hand vein punctures, the posterior, dorsal surface of the wrist is preferred because the veins are larger. It is not acceptable to puncture the anterior, or palmar, side. Nerves lie close to the palmar side and can easily be injured by needle probing. Also, on the palmar side, one can feel an artery pulsating. (p. 265)

35.

A. Arteries do not feel like veins. They have thicker vessel walls, pulsate, and are considered more elastic. (p. 267)

B. Veins are actually more blue in color.

C. Diameter of veins and arteries varies based on the location in the body.

D. The temperature of blood is the same in both arteries and veins.

36.

A.–D. (The correct answer is B.) Patients who have had mastectomies often have lymph nodes removed from the same surgical area. Swelling often occurs on the affected side of the body. Blood should not be withdrawn from the mastectomy side unless approved by a physician. However, the other arm should be considered first as an alternate site. (p. 268)

37.

A, C, D. The needle should never be inserted with the "bevel side down," with the "bevel pointed away from the insertion site," or "while perpendicular to the skin surface."

B. In a venipuncture procedure, the needle should always be inserted with the bevel side upward and directly above a prominent vein or slightly below the palpable vein. One can feel a slight "pop" as the needle enters the vein. (p. 273)

38.

A. Syringes do not cause excessive tissue fluid production.

B. Syringes are not routinely used for venipuncture because of needle safety concerns, and accidental cross-contamination of anticoagulants if the blood specimen is injected into multiple evacuated tubes using the same needle and syringe. (p. 275)

C. Needle size may vary widely when using a syringe. This is not the major concern.

D. The syringe method does not usually cause more pain than a routine venipuncture using the evacuated-tube method.

39.

A. Winged infusion sets are used for particularly difficult venipunctures. This includes patients with small hand or wrist veins, patients who are young children, patients who are severely burned, geriatric patients, patients who have had numerous needlesticks (such as oncology patients), patients in restrictive positions (arthritis), and those with fragile skin and veins. Young adult males usually have veins that are palpable and visible so a winged infusion set would not be as useful compared to the other situations described. (p. 275)

B, C, D. Winged infusion sets are used for particularly difficult venipunctures. This includes patients with small hand or wrist veins, patients who are young children, patients who are severely burned, geriatric patients, patients who have had numerous needlesticks (such as oncology patients), patients in restrictive positions (arthritis), and those with fragile skin and veins.

40.

A. Health care workers should be extra cautious as the needle is removed from the patient, and activating the safety device on the needle according to the manufacturer's instructions is the next step. There are varying methods of activating safety devices, so proper training and use are vital to keeping accidental needlesticks at a minimum. (p. 274)

B. Applying an adhesive bandage to the site is important toward the end of the encounter with the patient and after checking for bleeding. This is not the step immediately after needle withdrawal.

C. Labeling the specimen is also important toward the end of the encounter. This is not the step immediately after needle withdrawal.

D. Disposing of the needle and contaminated supplies is also important at the end of the encounter, but it is not the step immediately after needle withdrawal.

41.

A.–D. (The correct answer is D.) Clinical laboratories usually establish guidelines for specimen rejection. In general, the following factors are considered: improper transportation, hemolysis, anticoagulated specimens containing blood clots, inadequate volume in tube, unlabeled tubes, wrong collection tube, outdated supplies used, or visible contamination. (p. 282)

42.

A. The order of draw does not usually relate to proper filling.

B. Drawing the coagulation tubes after at least one other tube of blood diminishes the chances of contamination with tissue fluids, which may initiate the clotting sequence. However, recent studies suggest that accurate coagulation results may be obtained by using it as the first tube. Therefore, the phlebotomist must use the procedure specified by the health care facility. (p. 278)

C. The order of draw does not dictate the order that the tests will be performed in the laboratory.

D. The order of draw does not influence the status of the needle.

43.

A, B, C. The right volume of blood in the evacuated tube does not maintain homeostasis, prevent hemolysis, or promote bleeding.

D. The right volume of blood in the evacuated tube allows for the proper mix of anticoagulant-to-blood ratio. (p. 279)

44.

A. Forcefully mixing the specimen is not recommended and can cause the specimen to hemolyze.

B. Centrifugation is not an effective way to mix the anticoagulant with the blood.

C. Adequate mixing does not occur naturally during transportation.

D. Gentle inversion of the specimen after the procedure is needed to prevent the specimen from clotting. (p. 274)

45.

A. The most commonly requested timed specimen is for glucose level determinations, and is drawn 2 hours after a meal. (p. 282)

B. Cholesterol levels are not usually timed tests; however, fasting information is needed.

C. Triglyceride tests are not usually timed tests; however, fasting information is helpful.

D. Hemoglobin tests are commonly requested as part of the hematology tests ordered. However, it is not a timed test.

46.

A. Hormone levels increase and decrease depending on the time of day, so it is important to note the time of specimen collection; however, they are not monitored by drawing peak and trough specimens.

B. Peak and trough levels of certain drugs are useful to monitor the therapeutic levels. (p. 283)

C. Glucose screening is not referred to as "peak and trough levels."

D. Peak and trough levels are not related to gastric analysis.

47.

A. Safety devices on needles are not called butterflies.

B. An evacuated collection tube is not a butterfly.

C. A winged infusion set is often called a butterfly needle assembly. It is used for very small veins and/or particularly difficult veins. (p. 271)

D. The term "butterfly" does not refer to a syringe; however, a butterfly apparatus may be attached to a syringe.

48.

A. To minimize transfer of anticoagulants from one tube to the next, hold the tube horizontally or slightly downward during blood collection. This is more likely to keep the additive in one tube from coming into contact with the multisample needle, thereby reducing the risk of passing it on to the next tube. Cross-contamination of anticoagulants can cause erroneous results. (p. 279)

B. While specimen tubes should be treated carefully, this does not prevent the transfer of additives from one tube to the next.

C. A syringe method of transfer does, in fact, reduce the chances of cross-contamination with additives; however, this method is not recommended for routine use.

D. Drawing the coagulation tube first does not reduce the likelihood of cross-contamination of other additives.

49.

A. The earlobe would not be a suitable site for venipuncture or specimen acquisition for the amount of blood needed.

B. The heel of the foot should not be used in this case because of the risk of infections of the lower extremities in diabetics.

C. The posterior or dorsal side of the hand or wrist, below the site of the IV, could be used for venipuncture. The situation should be documented. (p. 268)

D. The anterior surface of the wrist should never be used for venipuncture.

50.

A. The preferred order of draw would be blood cultures, coagulation, hematology, and chemistry tubes. However, phlebotomists must follow the order of draw recommended by individual manufacturers and by their health care organizations. (p. 277)

B, C, D. These are not the "preferred order of draw"; however, phlebotomists should always follow their organization's procedures for the order of draw.

51.

A. A butterfly system could be used to diminish the likelihood of complications. In addition, the phlebotomist should be careful with site selection, and document the patient's condition to explain unusual results. (pp. 271–274)

B. A finger puncture would not suffice to collect enough blood for all the tests needed.

C. The phlebotomist should not decline to perform the procedure unless he has grave concerns about his own technical ability. However, most phlebotomists who work in a hospital situation are likely to encounter situations such as this one and should be prepared to use alternative methods.

D. A blood pressure cuff should not be tightened more than usual, especially since the arms are compromised with scarring, IVs, and/or fragile skin.

10 Procedures for Collecting Capillary Blood Specimens

chapter objectives

Upon completion of Chapter 10, the learner is responsible for the following:

➤ Describe reasons for acquiring capillary blood specimens.

➤ Identify the proper sites for performing a skin puncture procedure.

➤ Explain why controlling the depth of the incision is necessary.

➤ Describe the procedure for making a blood smear.

➤ Explain why capillary blood from a skin puncture procedure is different from blood taken by venipuncture.

DIRECTIONS Each of the questions or incomplete statements below is followed by four suggested answers or completions. Select one answer that is best in each case.

1. Alcohol that has not dried on a skin puncture can:
   A. prevent a round drop from forming
   B. facilitate making blood smears
   C. have a beneficial effect on laboratory tests
   D. provide an extra measure of sterility and reliability

2. Steps that are identical for venipuncture and finger-stick procedures are:
   A. site selection on fingers
   B. greeting, identification, and hand decontamination
   C. withdrawing the needle
   D. puncture technique

3. Skin puncture techniques are most often used when:
   A. small amounts of blood are needed for testing, as when the patient is a neonate or anemic
   B. the patient is normal but requires many routine blood tests
   C. the patient is an athelete and needs a drug screen
   D. routine microbiology tests are needed

4. Which of the following steps would *not* be part of a finger-stick procedure?
   A. The patient's finger should be held firmly.
   B. The puncture should be made in one sharp, continuous movement.
   C. Pressure should be applied to the puncture site to expel the blood.

   D. The puncture site can be selected from anywhere on the skin.

5. Refer to the photos in Figure 10.1. In the first photo, which is/are the preferred skin puncture sites?
   A. thumb
   B. pointer
   C. third and fourth fingers
   D. pinky finger

6. Refer to the second photo to answer this question. Which puncture is the preferred method for a finger stick?
   A. The side region of the finger labeled "A."
   B. The side region of the finger labeled "B."
   C. The second segment of the finger labeled "B."
   D. The fingertip region of the finger labeled "A."

7. Before a skin puncture procedure, a health care worker should do which of the following?
   A. emotional preparation
   B. supply and equipment preparation
   C. decontaminate hands and put on clean gloves
   D. all of the above

8. Capillary blood acquired by skin puncture is composed of:
   A. mostly arterial blood
   B. mostly venous blood
   C. mostly intracellular and interstitial fluids
   D. a combination of the above components listed in A, B, and C

FIGURE 10.1.

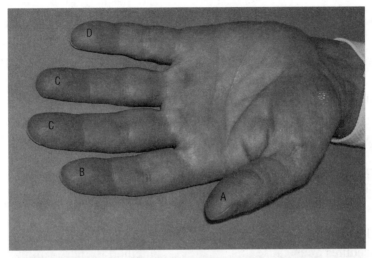

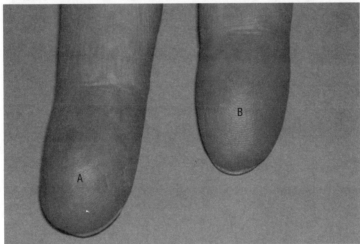

9. Fragile veins are most likely to be found in which type of patients?

   A. obese people

   B. people who do not exercise

   C. geriatric people

   D. teenagers

10. Capillary specimens are useful in which of the following situations?

    A. When veins are being "saved" for chemotherapy.

    B. When there are large quantities of blood needed for testing.

    C. When blood cultures are being collected.

    D. When hormone tests are being collected.

11. What is interstitial fluid?

    A. synovial fluid

    B. capillary blood

    C. spinal fluid

    D. tissue fluid

12. Why is venipuncture more hazardous for small children?
    A. It is not more hazardous for children than for adults.
    B. It makes children more likely to develop allergies.
    C. It increases risks of anemia and infections.
    D. It increases risks of blood disorders.

13. Which reason explains how a venipuncture can cause anemia?
    A. Too much blood is withdrawn.
    B. The procedure can be traumatic.
    C. The patient's anxiety can cause this problem.
    D. The decontamination process can cause this problem.

14. Labeled skin puncture specimens should include the:
    A. patient's name and identification number
    B. time and date of collection
    C. phlebotomist's initials
    D. all of the above

15. Which of the following conditions can have an adverse effect on the quality of a finger stick?
    A. the age of a patient
    B. the gender of a patient
    C. using the first drop of blood
    D. the presence of a wedding ring

16. Blood smears for evaluation of cells must be made carefully. Which of the following features should not be present?
    A. one half of the slide being covered
    B. a feathered edge
    C. ridges and holes in the smear
    D. even, thin layer of blood

17. Skin puncture blood is composed of:
    A. tissue fluids
    B. blood from arterioles and venules
    C. blood from capillaries
    D. a combination of A, B, and C

18. Skin puncture samples are often used for which of the following tests?
    A. white blood cell differentials
    B. blood cultures
    C. blood gases
    D. therapeutic drug levels

19. Which of the listed sequences is the best method for performing a finger stick?
    A. Squeeze the finger, decontaminate, puncture the skin.
    B. Decontaminate, squeeze the finger, puncture the skin, collect the first drop.
    C. Decontaminate, puncture the skin, wipe the first drop, collect the sample.
    D. Apply tourniquet, puncture the skin, wipe the first drop, collect the sample.

20. Warming a site for skin puncture:
    A. increases blood pressure
    B. increases blood flow to the site
    C. relaxes the patient
    D. eliminates the need for a tourniquet

21. What should the phlebotomist do with the first drop of blood after a finger stick is performed?
    A. Use it for coagulation studies.
    B. Make a blood smear or slide.
    C. Wipe it off with gauze.
    D. Use it for hematology testing.

22. Which of the following facilitate site preparation for skin puncture?
    A. commercially available warming devices
    B. preheated tubes
    C. ice water
    D. gauze

23. What is the best angle for spreading a blood smear by using two glass slides?
    A. 15 degrees
    B. 30 degrees
    C. 45 degrees
    D. 60 degrees

24. Normally, which of the following should be used to decontaminate the site before skin puncture?
    A. isopropanol
    B. povidone-iodine
    C. diluted chlorox
    D. methanol

25. What is the average depth a skin puncture should be for an adult?
    A. 0.5 to 1.0 mm
    B. 2 to 3 mm
    C. 3 to 5 mm
    D. 5–7 mm

26. Excessive massaging or milking of the finger during a skin puncture procedure can cause:
    A. an adequate supply of blood for filling several capillary tubes
    B. increased venous blood flow to the puncture site
    C. hemolysis and contamination of the specimen with tissue fluids
    D. better results for glucose screening

27. Osteomyelitis is defined as:
    A. infection of the blood
    B. infection of the spinal fluid
    C. infection of the bone
    D. infection of the finger

28. How does a capillary tube fill with blood during a skin puncture procedure?
    A. using suction from the collection device
    B. using the vacuum in the tube
    C. blood flows freely into the tube on contact
    D. gravity pulls the blood down into the tube

29. In making a blood smear or slide, after the drop of blood has been spread across the glass slide, what is the next step?
    A. Gently blow on it to aid in drying.
    B. Hold it over a heating element to promote cellular adhesion to the glass.
    C. Add a drop of saline to the slide to preserve it.
    D. Allow it to air-dry.

30. What can happen if an EDTA microcollection tube is overfilled?
    A. Clots may form in the tube.
    B. The patient is likely to faint.
    C. The tests will be falsely negative.
    D. Cell morphology may change.

31. What can happen if an EDTA microcollection tube is underfilled?
    A. Clots may form in the tube.
    B. The patient is likely to faint.
    C. The tests will be falsely negative.
    D. Cell morphology may change.

32. Should glass capillary tubes be avoided?
    A. Yes, because they break easily.
    B. Yes, because they hurt the patient.
    C. No, they are safe and effective.
    D. No, they are economical and easy to handle.

33. When is "fasting" an important consideration for collecting capillary specimens?
    A. It is only an important factor for collecting capillary specimens from the elderly.
    B. It is an important factor for collecting many capillary specimens.
    C. It is irrelevant and has no effect on capillary specimens.
    D. It is only an important factor when testing for glucose.

34. What effect does dehydration have on skin puncture?
    A. If a patient is dehydrated, it has no effect on skin puncture.
    B. If a patient is dehydrated, bleeding may be more difficult.
    C. If a patient is dehydrated, he/she is more likely to bleed excessively.
    D. If a patient is dehydrated, she is more likely to perspire.

35. Why is the earlobe not a "preferred site" for skin puncture?
    A. It has more nerves than other places on the body.
    B. It is close to the bone.
    C. It may cause anxiety due to the close proximity to the eyes.
    D. It is more easily bruised.

36. Which of the following are *not* recommended sites for skin puncture?
    A. third finger of an adult
    B. third or fourth finger of a newborn
    C. the fourth finger of an adult
    D. heel of an infant

37. What is another term for PCV?
    A. pediatric cell volume
    B. hematocrit or packed cell volume
    C. pediatric cellular velocity
    D. hemoglobin value

38. Which of the following fingers has a "pulse"?
    A. pinky finger
    B. pointer finger
    C. middle finger
    D. thumb

39. Identify the skin puncture device that is an alternative to a retractable lancet.
    A. radio frequency lance
    B. scantag
    C. laser
    D. metallic clip

40. What type of lancet is most often recommended for skin puncture?
    A. nonretractable
    B. retractable
    C. puncture proof
    D. surgical knife

41. The "order of draw" for filling microcollection tubes with capillary blood is:
    A. the same as for venipunctures
    B. not the same as for venipunctures

C. the same as when using the butterfly method

D. the same as for IV therapy

42. What is the appropriate order of filling microcollection tubes with capillary blood from the *first* drop of blood expelled from the finger?

A. EDTA specimen for hematology tests, other tubes with additives, nonadditive tubes

B. additive tubes, then nonadditive tubes

C. coagulation tubes, then nonadditive tubes

D. This procedure is not appropriate for filling tubes.

43. What is the appropriate order of filling microcollection tubes with capillary blood from the second drop of blood expelled from the finger?

A. EDTA specimen for hematology tests, other tubes with additives, nonadditive tubes

B. blood cultures, then nonadditive tubes

C. coagulation tubes, then nonadditive tubes

D. This procedure is not appropriate for filling tubes.

44. How should used lancets be disposed?

A. puncture-proof trash can

B. puncture-proof biohazard sharps container

C. They should be transported to the nearest laboratory and discarded.

D. They should be placed in alcohol and then reused.

45. Which statement describes a "cyanotic" finger?

A. bluish in color due to insufficient oxygen

B. yellow in color due to liver failure

C. green in color due to infection

D. swollen

46. During a skin puncture procedure, how should the cut be oriented on the finger?

A. on a diagonal

B. parallel to the fingerprint lines

C. across the fingerprint lines

D. It doesn't matter how the lancet is positioned, it is done automatically.

47. After a skin puncture procedure, where should the phlebotomist dispose of contaminated gloves?

A. in the trash can located at the patient's bedside

B. in a biohazard container

C. They should be transported to the laboratory and disposed of with other lab trash.

D. Gloves should be taken to the nursing station for proper disposal.

48. How should the phlebotomist treat a microcollection tube with additives once the blood specimen is taken?

A. It should be shaken vigorously.

B. It should be frozen.

C. It should be shaken gently.

D. It should be placed in a heating block.

49. Air bubbles in microcollection tubes can do which of the following?

A. assist in blood flow

B. keep the blood from spilling out of the tube

C. cause delayed clotting

D. cause erroneous results

50. What procedure is needed when collecting capillary blood for blood gases?

   A. cooling the site

   B. warming the site

   C. sticking deeper into the skin

   D. using a special arterial lancet

51. What is the last step in any phlebotomy procedure, including skin puncture?

   A. Make blood smears.

   B. Apply pressure to the site.

   C. Label specimens.

   D. Check that the bleeding has stopped and thank the patient for cooperating.

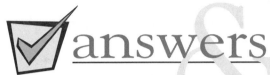answers & rationales

1.

A. The skin puncture site should be cleaned with 70% isopropanol and thoroughly dried before being punctured because residual alcohol prevents round drops of blood from forming, which is needed for blood smear preparation. (p. 293)

B. Excess alcohol does not facilitate making blood smears.

C. Residual alcohol does not have a beneficial effect on laboratory results.

D. While residual alcohol may, in fact, provide an extra measure of sterility, it does not provide an extra measure of test reliability.

2.

A. Site selection is different for the two procedures.

B. Steps that are identical for venipuncture and skin puncture procedures are greeting, identification, and hand-washing. (p. 291)

C. Withdrawing the needle is different for the two procedures, especially in the types of supplies and physical maneuvers that are required by the phlebotomist.

D. The puncture technique is also different for the two procedures in that timing, feel/touch, and application of pressure vary significantly.

3.

A. Skin puncture techniques are most often used when small amounts of blood are needed for testing, when a patient is anemic, or complications may exist such as cardiac arrest, hemorrhage, venous thrombosis, reflex arteriospasm, gangrene of an extremity, danger to surrounding tissues or organs, infections, and injuries from restraining a child. Skin punctures are useful if the patient is a neonate, infant, or small child. (p. 290)

B. Skin puncture techniques are not often used when the patient requires many routine blood tests.

C. Skin puncture techniques are not often used when the patient is an athlete and needs drug screening.

D. Skin puncture techniques are not often used when microbiology tests are needed.

4.

A.–C. The finger-stick procedure involves holding a patient's finger firmly with the phlebotomist's thumb away from the puncture site. The puncture should be done in one sharp, continuous movement, and gentle pressure can be applied to the finger.

D. The finger-stick procedure involves holding a patient's finger firmly with the phlebotomist's thumb away from the puncture site. The puncture should be done in one sharp, continuous movement, and gentle pressure can be applied to the finger. The preferred sites for skin puncture are the third or fourth finger. (pp. 296–297)

5.

A. The thumb is not a preferred site for skin puncture. Positioning of the hand can be more awkward.

B. The pointer finger is not the preferred site.

C. Preferred skin puncture sites are the fleshy portion of the third and fourth fingers. (p. 293)

D. The pinky finger is not recommended for skin puncture because the tissue of this finger is thinner than that of the others.

FIGURE 10.1. Sites for finger puncture.

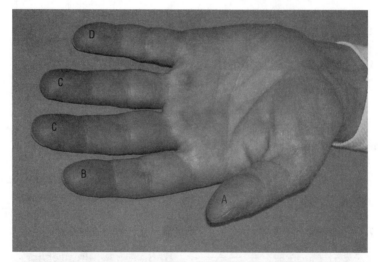

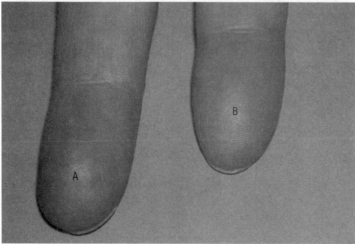

6.

A.–B. The side regions of fingers are not preferred sites because the tissue is not as thick and there is a higher risk of hitting a bone when punctured.

C. The second segment of the finger is not a preferred site.

D. The preferred site is the fleshy, central surface of the fingertip (not the extreme tip) on the third finger. (pp. 292–293)

7.

A.–D. (The correct answer is D.) Before performing a skin puncture, the health care worker should prepare him- or herself emotionally for the encounter, choose needed supplies and equipment, wash hands and put on clean gloves, and continue with the appropriate identification and greetings of the patient. (p. 291)

8.

A.–D. (The correct answer is D.) Capillary blood acquired by skin puncture is significantly different than that of venous blood acquired by venipuncture. It is composed of blood from arteries, venules, capillaries, and intracellular and interstitial fluids. (p. 290)

9.

A. Obese patients do not normally have fragile veins.

B. Lack of exercise does not normally contribute to having fragile veins.

C. Geriatric patients are likely to have fragile veins. (p. 290)

D. Teenagers do not normally have fragile veins.

10.

A. Capillary specimens are useful when veins are being saved for chemotherapy in oncology patients. (p. 290)

B. When large quantities of blood are needed for testing, capillary specimens are not useful.

C. Capillary specimens are not recommended for blood cultures.

D. Capillary specimens are not recommended for hormone tests.

11.

A. Synovial fluid is fluid found in between joints; it is not interstitial fluid.

B. Capillary blood is not interstitial fluid even though it is partially composed of interstitial fluid.

C. Spinal fluid is not interstitial fluid.

D. Interstitial fluid is "tissue" fluid. (p. 290)

12.

A. Venipuncture *is* more hazardous for children because of the increased risk of complications.

B. Venipuncture does not normally cause children to develop allergies.

C. Venipuncture is more hazardous for children because of the increased risk of complications such as anemia and infections. (p. 290)

D. Venipuncture does not increase risks of blood disorders.

13.

A. When too much blood is withdrawn from a small child or infant, the blood volume may be significantly reduced. (p. 290)

B. Venipuncture is usually minimally traumatic but it would not cause anemia.

C. The patient's anxiety would not cause anemia.

D. The decontamination process would not cause anemia.

14.

A.–D. (The correct answer is D.) Labeled skin puncture specimens should include the same information as on a venipuncture specimen, including the patient's name and identification number, the time and date of collection, and the phlebotomist's initials. (p. 291)

15.

A. The age of a patient does not have an adverse effect on a skin puncture, even though the health care worker needs to consider special circumstances in dealing with elderly patients.

B. The gender of a patient does not have an adverse effect on a skin puncture.

C. Using the first drop of blood can have an adverse effect on a skin puncture specimen because it may be diluted with tissue fluids, thus causing erroneous results in laboratory tests. (p. 296)

D. The presence of a wedding ring will not have an adverse effect on a skin puncture.

16.

A. Good blood smears should cover about one half of the slide.

B. Good blood smears have a feathered edge.

C. No ridges, lines, or holes should be present on a blood smear. (p. 300)

D. Blood smears should have an even, thin layer of blood.

17.

A.–D. (The correct answer is D.) Skin puncture blood is composed of tissue fluids, blood from arterioles and venules, and blood from capillaries. The content of arterial blood is actually greater in skin puncture blood than of venous blood because the arterial pressure in the capillaries is stronger than the venous pressure. (p. 290)

18.

A. Skin puncture samples are often used for white blood cell differentials. They are also used for a variety of screening tests (e.g., glucose, cholesterol) and other point-of-care procedures. (p. 295)

B. Blood cultures are performed by venipuncture to minimize contamination and to acquire the amount of blood needed for detection of the infectious microorganisms.

C. Blood gases are usually evaluated using arterial samples.

D. Drug levels usually require urine or larger amounts of blood than are possible from a skin puncture.

19.

A. The following steps are *not* in the correct order. Squeeze the finger, decontaminate, puncture the skin.

B. The following steps are *not* in the correct order: Decontaminate, squeeze the finger, puncture the skin, collect the first drop. Also, the first drop should be wiped off before collecting the sample.

C. The best method for performing a finger stick involves decontaminating the site, puncturing the skin, wiping the first drop, and collecting the sample. (pp. 296–297)

D. A tourniquet is not necessary in a skin puncture procedure.

20.

A. Warming a site for skin puncture does not increase blood pressure.

B. Warming a site for skin puncture increases blood flow to the site. (p. 292)

C. Warming a site for skin puncture does not necessarily relax the patient.

D. Warming a site for skin puncture has nothing to do with the need for a tourniquet, since tourniquets are not used for skin puncture procedures.

21.

A. The first drop of blood is not generally recommended for coagulation studies because it is mixed with tissue fluids.

B. The first drop of blood is not generally recommended for making a blood smear or slide because it is mixed with tissue fluids, so the blood is actually somewhat diluted.

C. After a finger stick is performed, the phlebotomist should wipe off the first drop of blood. (p. 296)

D. The first drop of blood is not generally recommended for hematology testing.

22.

A. Commercially available warming devices can facilitate site preparation. (p. 292)

B. Preheated tubes do not facilitate site preparation.

C. Ice water does not facilitate site preparation.

D. Gauze does not facilitate site preparation.

23.

A. 15 degrees is incorrect.

B. The best angle for spreading a blood smear using two glass slides is approximately 30 degrees. (p. 299)

C. 45 degrees is incorrect.

D. 60 degrees is incorrect.

24.

A. Isopropanol should be used to decontaminate the site before skin puncture. (pp. 296–297)

B. Povidone-iodine may be used to decontaminate skin puncture sites under special circumstances; however, isopropanol is the recommended choice.

C. Diluted chlorox is not a recommended decontaminating agent for skin.

D. Methanol is not a recommended decontaminating agent for skin.

25.

A. A puncture depth of 0.5 to 1.0 mm may be too shallow to get adequate blood flowing for sample collection.

B. The average depth of a skin puncture should be 2 to 3 mm for an adult to avoid hitting the bone. (p. 294)

C. A puncture depth of 3 to 5 mm is too deep and may puncture the bone; this could lead to complications such as osteomyelitis.

D. A puncture depth of 5–7 mm is hazardous to the patient for the reasons mentioned above.

26.

A. Gentle massaging of the finger can assist in providing an adequate supply of blood for filling several capillary tubes; however, excessive massaging can damage the cells.

B. Excessive massaging or milking of the finger does not increase venous blood flow to the puncture site.

C. Excessive massaging or milking of the finger during a skin puncture procedure can cause hemolysis and contamination of the specimen with tissue fluids. (pp. 296–297)

D. Excessive massaging or milking of the finger does not achieve better results in glucose screening tests; rather, it can cause erroneous results.

27.

A. Sepsis is an infection of the blood.

B. Meningitis is an infection of the spinal cord, fluid, and meninges.

C. Osteomyelitis is defined as inflammation and infection of the bone. (p. 294)

D. There is no specific term for an infection of the finger.

28.

A. It is not necessary to use suction from the collection device when filling capillary tubes.

B. There is no vacuum in capillary tubes.

C. A capillary tube fills with blood during a skin puncture procedure using capillary action, whereby blood flows freely into the tube on contact without suction. (pp. 296–297)

D. Capillary tubes do not require a downward position (for gravity to have an influence). However, blood flow from the finger may be better if the puncture site is held downward and gentle pressure is applied.

29.

A. Blood smears should never be blown on to aid in drying.

B. Blood smears should never be held over a heating element to promote cellular adhesion to the glass because cells may be destroyed in the process.

C. Blood smears do not require saline to preserve the cells.

D. In making a blood smear or slide, after the drop of blood has been spread across the glass slide, the next step is to allow it to air-dry and label it. (p. 299)

30.

A. Overfilling of an EDTA microcollection tube can cause clot formation. (p. 298)

B. The patient is not likely to faint due to overfilling.

C. Tests will not be falsely negative due to overfilling.

D. Cell morphology is not likely to change due to overfilling.

31.

A. Clots are not likely to form in the tube.

B. The patient is not likely to faint due to underfilling.

C. Tests will not be falsely negative due to overfilling.

D. Cell morphology may change because of inadequate filling, thereby altering the blood to additive ratio (i.e., too much anticoagulant in the tube). (p. 298)

32.

A. Phlebotomists are at risk of injury if glass capillary tubes shatter. Regulatory agencies have recommended the use of devices that are less likely to break. (p. 292)

B. Glass capillary tubes do not normally hurt the patient.

C. Glass capillary tubes are not as safe or effective as nonglass tubes.

D. While glass capillary tubes are economical and easy to handle, they should be avoided due to safety concerns.

33.

A. Fasting is an important consideration for all types of patients.

B. Fasting status is important for collecting many types of blood specimens. (p. 291)

C. Fasting status is *not* irrelevant.

D. Fasting is an important consideration for many types of laboratory tests.

34.

A. If a patient is dehydrated, it does have an effect on skin puncture.

B. If a patient is dehydrated, bleeding may be more difficult because the blood volume is lower. It may require warming the site and giving the patient something to drink. (p. 290)

C. If a patient is dehydrated, she is not more likely to bleed excessively.

D. If a patient is dehydrated, she is not more likely to perspire.

35.

A. The earlobe does not have more nerves than other places on the body.

B. The earlobe is not close to the bone

C. Using the earlobe for skin puncture is still in practice by some phlebotomists; however it is not preferred due to possible interference with pierced earrings and the close proximity to the eyes (which may cause undue anxiety). (p. 294)

D. The earlobe does not bruise more easily than other sites.

36.

A. The third finger of an adult is an acceptable site for skin puncture.

B. The fingers of newborns are not recommended for skin puncture sites. (p. 294)

C. The fourth finger of an adult is an acceptable site for skin puncture.

D. The heel of an infant is an acceptable site for skin puncture.

37.

A. Pediatric cell volume is not another term for PCV.

B. Hematocrit or packed cell volume is another term for PCV. (p. 295)

C. Pediatric cellular velocity is not another term for PCV.

D. Hemoglobin value is not another term for PCV.

38.

A. The pinky finger does not have a pulse.

B. The pointer finger does not have a pulse.

C. The middle finger does not have a pulse.

D. The thumb does have a pulse. (p. 294)

39.

A. Radio frequency lance is not an appropriate answer.

B. Scantag is not an appropriate answer.

C. Laser devices are skin puncture alternatives. (p. 294)

D. A metallic clip is not an appropriate answer.

40.

A. Nonretractable lancets are not most often recommended for skin puncture.

B. Retractable lancets are most often recommended for skin puncture. (p. 295)

C. Puncture proof lancets are not most often recommended for skin puncture.

D. Surgical knives are not most often recommended for skin puncture.

41.

A. The "order of draw" for filling microcollection tubes with capillary blood is not the same as for venipunctures.

B. The "order of draw" for filling microcollection tubes with capillary blood is not the same as for venipunctures. (p. 295)

C. The "order of draw" for filling microcollection tubes with capillary blood is not the same as when using a butterfly method.

D. This answer is not appropriate.

42.

A.–D. (The correct answer is D.) Using the first drop of blood is not appropriate for filling any tubes. The first drop should always be wiped off and the collection procedure should begin with the second drop. (pp. 296–297)

43.

A. The appropriate order of filling microcollection tubes with capillary blood from the second drop of blood expelled from the finger is EDTA specimen for hematology tests, other tubes with additives, nonadditive tubes. (p. 295)

B, C, D. These are not appropriate responses.

44.

A. Lancets should not be placed in a trash can.

B. Used lancets should be immediately discarded into a puncture-proof biohazard sharps container. (p. 295)

C and D. Used lancets should not be transported or placed in alcohol and reused, they should be discarded immediately in the appropriate container.

45.

A. A cyanotic finger is bluish in color due to insufficient oxygen. (p. 296)

B. A cyanotic finger is not yellow.

C. A cyanotic finger is not green.

D. A cyanotic finger is not necessarily swollen.

46.

A. During the skin puncture procedure, the cut should not be oriented on the diagonal.

B. During the skin puncture procedure, the cut should not be oriented parallel to the fingerprint lines.

C. During the skin puncture procedure, the cut should be oriented across the fingerprint lines. (pp. 296–297)

D. This answer is inappropriate.

47.

A. Gloves should not be thrown into the trash.

B. Contaminated gloves should be disposed of in a biohazardous container adjacent to the procedure area. (p. 297)

C. Gloves should not be transported. They should be disposed of immediately.

D. Gloves should not be taken to the nursing station for disposal. They should be disposed of immediately.

48.

A. Specimens should never be shaken vigorously.

B. Specimens should not be frozen unless there are special circumstances.

C. Specimens should be gently inverted to mix the additive with the blood. (p. 297)

D. Specimens should not be placed in a heating block unless there are special circumstances.

49.

A. Air bubbles in microcollection tubes do not assist in blood flow.

B. Air bubbles in microcollection tubes do not keep the blood from spilling out of the tube.

C. Air bubbles in microcollection tubes do not cause delayed clotting.

D. Air bubbles in microcollection tubes can cause erroneous laboratory results. (p. 297)

50.

A. Cooling the site is not appropriate.

B. Warming the site increases arterial blood flow to the area. (p. 298)

C. Sticking deeper into the skin is not an acceptable practice.

D. This answer is not appropriate.

51.

A. Making blood smears is often one of the final phases in the procedure; however, it is not always the last.

B. Applying pressure to the site is one of the final phases in the procedure, however, it is not always the last.

C. Labeling specimens is one of the final phases in the procedure; however, it is not always the last.

D. Ensuring that the bleeding has stopped and thanking the patient for their cooperation should be the final step in any blood collection procedure. (p. 297)

11 Preanalytical Complications in Blood Collection

chapter objectives

Upon completion of Chapter 11, the learner is responsible for the following:

➤ Describe preanalytical complications related to phlebotomy.

➤ Explain how to prevent and/or handle complications in blood collection.

➤ List at least five factors about a patient's physical disposition that can affect blood collection.

➤ List examples of substances that can interfere in the clinical analysis of blood constituents and describe methods used to prevent these interferences.

DIRECTIONS Each of the questions or incomplete statements below is followed by four suggested answers or completions. Select one answer that is best in each case.

1. What does the term "preanalytical" refer to in phlebotomy practice?
   A. equipment malfunction during testing
   B. variables that affect the specimen prior to laboratory analysis
   C. an episode of syncope
   D. when a test result is reported incorrectly

2. What is the ideal time for specimens to be collected?
   A. at midnight
   B. 5 hours after the last ingestion of food
   C. 12 hours after the last ingestion of food
   D. 24 hours after the last ingestion of food

3. Why is it important to collect blood when the patient is in a basal state?
   A. Because it is most comfortable for the patient at this time.
   B. Because laboratory tests are most reliable if the patient is in a basal state.
   C. Because blood is thickest at this time.
   D. Because it fits well into the preestablished work schedules of most hospitals.

4. What happens if a patient abstains from drinking water for 12–24 hours?
   A. Nothing happens, this is a standard procedure for all hospitals.
   B. The specimen will be somewhat diluted.
   C. The patient may become dehydrated.
   D. The glucose level would be elevated.

5. How many adults in the United States are overweight?
   A. less than 10%
   B. 20%
   C. more than 50%
   D. 100%

6. If a patient asks to chew sugarless gum prior to a "fasting glucose" procedure, what should the phlebotomist say?
   A. The phlebotomist should say that it is okay to chew sugarless gum.
   B. The phlebotomist should explain that chewing gum may cause a transient fluctuation in the blood sugar level.
   C. The phlebotomist should say it is okay to have coffee or tea but not gum.
   D. The phlebotomist should advise the patient to chew the gum only for 5 minutes.

7. If a patient is overweight and the phlebotomist cannot access the vein when the needle is first inserted, what should the phlebotomist do?
   A. Repalpate and adjust/move the needle very slightly.
   B. Probe around until the vein is found.
   C. Push the needle all the way in because the vein is probably under layers of fat.
   D. Give up the procedure and allow someone else to do it.

8. What effect does excessive probing with a needle in the patient's arm have on a venipuncture specimen?
   A. No effect at all and the specimen should be acceptable.
   B. It can rupture RBCs and release clotting factors.
   C. Probing is often necessary and only alters the WBC count.
   D. No effect, but a physician should be notified of the circumstances.

9. What effects do prolonged fasting or severe diets have on patients?
   A. No effects at all.
   B. Only glucose tolerance levels are affected.
   C. Only RBC counts are affected.
   D. Electrolyte disturbances and cardiac dysrhythmias may result.

10. What does the term "occluded" mean in relation to veins?
    A. larger than normal
    B. smaller than normal
    C. obstructed
    D. inflamed due to an infection

11. If a patient is allergic to iodine and alcohol, what could be used to disinfect the puncture site?
    A. chlorox
    B. chlorohexidine
    C. acetone
    D. soap and water

12. Effects of exercise on laboratory tests are dependent on which factors?
    A. intensity and duration of the exercise
    B. frequency of doing the exercise

    C. gender and age
    D. all of the above

13. What does the term "edema" mean?
    A. obesity
    B. infection of the skin
    C. renal failure
    D. buildup of fluid

14. What is the most common cause of iron-deficiency anemia in women?
    A. excessive blood loss due to phlebotomy
    B. hemorrhage
    C. renal failure
    D. menstrual blood loss

15. In *most* cases, when should blood be collected to determine blood levels of medications?
    A. at 7:00 AM
    B. at 10:00 AM
    C. 30 minutes after the medication is administered
    D. just prior to the next dose of the medication

16. Which of the following analytes is significantly increased in the blood with changes in position?
    A. testosterone
    B. glucose
    C. cortisol
    D. iron

17. A solid mass derived from blood constituents that occlude a blood vessel is/are:
    A. lymphostasis
    B. angiography
    C. thrombi
    D. petechiae

18. If blood is to be collected for a timed blood glucose level determination, the patient must fast for:
    A. 4–6 hours
    B. 6–8 hours
    C. 8–12 hours
    D. 14–16 hours

19. Which of the following laboratory test results are affected most if the specimen is exposed to light for one hour?
    A. cortisol
    B. bilirubin
    C. testosterone
    D. CPK

20. Emotional stress, such as anxiety or fear of blood collections, can lead to an increase in:
    A. blood glucose
    B. RBC count
    C. WBC count
    D. serum iron

21. What effect does hyperventilation have on laboratory values?
    A. increased blood glucose
    B. increased cell counts
    C. increased serum iron
    D. acid-base imbalances

22. Upon entering Mrs. Martinez's hospital room, the phlebotomist noticed that Mrs. Martinez was taking three aspirin tablets. The patient commented that she was taking a second dose of aspirin because the first dose she took last night did not help her headache. What blood test will most likely be affected by the aspirin intake?
    A. triglycerides
    B. glucose

C. RBC count
D. platelet function tests

23. If the tourniquet is incorrectly applied for longer than 3 minutes, which of the following blood analytes will most likely become falsely elevated?
    A. uric acid
    B. blood urea nitrogen
    C. potassium
    D. bilirubin

24. A basal state exists:
    A. after the evening meal
    B. in the early morning, 12 hours after the last ingestion of food
    C. in the afternoon, 3 hours after ingestion of lunch
    D. before lunch

25. The phlebotomist assigned to collect a blood specimen from Ms. Smiley noticed that her right arm was swollen. She had recently had a mastectomy. This abnormal accumulation of fluid in the intercellular spaces of the body that is localized or diffused is referred to as:
    A. edema
    B. atherosclerosis
    C. hemolysis
    D. hemoconcentration

26. During a venipuncture procedure, when the area around a venipuncture site starts to swell, this occurrence usually leads to:
    A. atherosclerosis
    B. lymphostasis
    C. hematoma formation
    D. petechiae formation

27. Which of the following blood analytes is affected by diurnal rhythm?
    A. ACTH
    B. CK
    C. cholesterol
    D. creatinine

28. When the phlebotomist collected blood from the patient, the patient was in a supine position. This means the patient was:
    A. sitting on a chair
    B. lying on his stomach
    C. lying on his back
    D. standing near a counter

29. The phlebotomist went to Mr. Howell's hospital room to collect blood. The patient had already been transported to the cardiology unit for angiography. When the phlebotomist arrived at the cardiology unit, the patient had already undergone the angiography procedure. What blood laboratory test would be erroneously affected by the angiography procedure?
    A. creatinine and cortisol
    B. reticulocyte count
    C. RBC count
    D. WBC count

30. Which of the following blood analytes increases with age?
    A. growth hormone
    B. estrogen
    C. cholesterol and triglycerides
    D. bilirubin

31. Another term for fainting is:
    A. syncope
    B. lymphostasis
    C. transient blood
    D. thrombus

32. What does the term "falsely decreased" laboratory result refer to?
    A. A laboratory result that is interpreted as subnormal even though the blood analyte is truly in an elevated range or normal range.
    B. A laboratory result that is erroneously interpreted as normal
    C. A laboratory result caused by increasing the color produced in the laboratory test.
    D. A laboratory result that does not have a significant impact on the patient's outcome.

33. Which of the following should stop the health care worker from collecting blood from a patient's arm vein?
    A. high blood pressure
    B. cardiac bypass surgery
    C. heart attack that occurred the previous night
    D. mastectomy

34. Which of the following has been shown to erroneously affect laboratory test results, leading to falsely elevated or decreased results?
    A. smiling
    B. violent crying
    C. syncope
    D. sneezing

35. If a patient becomes extremely anxious and stressed during the blood collection procedure and begins to hyperventilate, which of the following laboratory results will become altered because of this stress?
    A. triglyceride level
    B. RBC count
    C. protein level
    D. blood pH level

FIGURE 11.1.

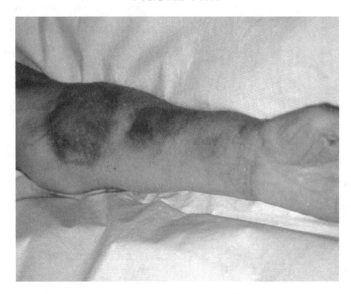

Source: Johnson & Johnson Medical Division, Ethicon, Inc., 1997. Used with permission of the copyright owner.

36. Which of the following would most likely *not* be an explanation for turbid serum?
    A. elevated triglyceride results
    B. elevated cholesterol results
    C. bacterial contamination
    D. elevated glucose results

37. What does Figure 11.1 depict?
    A. a hematoma appearing close to the antecubital fossa area
    B. a woman's arm showing lymphostasis
    C. petechiae close to the antecubital
    D. a woman's arm showing hemoconcentration

38. Which of the following occurs as the result of repeated punctures, inflammation, and disease of the interstitial compartments?
    A. hematoma
    B. hemoconcentration
    C. sclerosed veins
    D. syncope

39. "Falsely increased" laboratory results for a blood analyte is which of the following conditions?
    A. Results are interpreted as normal but the blood analyte is truly in an elevated range
    B. Results caused by a medication competing with the blood analyte for a chromogenic reagent, thus falsely decreasing the resultant color of the reaction.
    C. Results are interpreted as elevated but the blood analyte is truly in a normal range or a decreased range.
    D. The laboratory results are insignificant.

40. When hemoglobin is released and serum becomes tinged with pink or red, this condition is referred to as:
    A. lymphocytosis
    B. hemoconcentration
    C. hemolysis
    D. hemophilia

41. If the phlebotomist is preparing to collect specimens for routine hematology, coagulation, and chemistry tests, and notices that the patient is taking aspirin, why should the phlebotomist be concerned?
    A. Because the patient may bleed excessively.
    B. Because the BUN will be erroneous.
    C. Because the H and H will be altered.
    D. There is no cause for concern.

42. If the phlebotomist is preparing to collect specimens for routine hematology, coagulation, and chemistry tests, and notices that the patient is on IV heparin therapy, why should the phlebotomist be concerned?
    A. Because the patient may bleed excessively.
    B. Because the BUN will be erroneous.
    C. Because the H and H will be altered.
    D. There is no cause for concern.

43. If the phlebotomist is preparing to collect specimens for routine hematology, coagulation, and chemistry tests, and notices that the patient is on IV Warfarin, why should the phlebotomist be concerned?
    A. Because the patient may bleed excessively.
    B. Because the BUN will be erroneous.
    C. Because the H and H will be altered.
    D. There is no cause for concern.

44. What is the effect on a patient if a phlebotomist punctures a nerve with the phlebotomy needle?
    A. It should not have an effect on the patient.
    B. It may tingle slightly but it should not interfere with the rest of the procedure.
    C. The specimen may be contaminated with interstitial fluid.
    D. The patient will feel a sharp radiating pain and the procedure should be discontinued.

45. How long after a venipuncture procedure should pressure be applied to the puncture site?
    A. 30 seconds
    B. 60 seconds
    C. 90 seconds
    D. until the bleeding has stopped

46. Which of the following laboratory results will deteriorate rapidly if the specimen to be tested is not chilled?
    A. RBC
    B. WBC
    C. sickle cells
    D. ammonia

47. If a phlebotomist collects a venipuncture specimen from an arm site slightly above the patient's IV (in the same arm), what effect does it have on the specimen?
    A. No effect.
    B. It will increase the cellular counts.
    C. It will increase ammonia levels.
    D. It will dilute the specimen with IV fluids.

48. Identify the primary cause of "vein collapse" during venipuncture.
    A. Blood is withdrawn too quickly or forcefully.
    B. The tourniquet is not tight enough.
    C. The tourniquet is too tight.
    D. The tube has no vacuum in it.

49. CLSI suggests that cells be removed/separated from serum or plasma how long after collection?
    A. 15 minutes
    B. 1 hour
    C. 2 hours
    D. 12 hours

50. What is "room temperature"?
    A. 4 degrees Celsuis
    B. 15 degrees Celsius
    C. 22 degrees Celsius
    D. 75 degrees Celsius

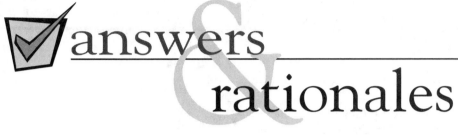
answers & rationales

1.

A. An equipment malfunction is an "analytical" variable.

B. In phlebotomy practice the term "preanalytical" refers to what happens to the specimen prior to laboratory analysis. Preanalytical variables can be controlled by the phlebotomist to minimize the risk of complications during or after the venipuncture procedure. (p. 304)

C. Syncope is one possible complication of phlebotomy; however, it does not normally have an effect on laboratory results.

D. An erroneous test result would be an example of a post-analytical event.

2.

A. Midnight is not the ideal time for specimen collection.

B. The ideal time for specimens to be collected is in the early morning, approximately 12 hours after the last ingestion of food.

C. The ideal time for specimens to be collected is in the early morning, approximately 12 hours after the last ingestion of food. (p. 304)

D. The ideal time for specimens to be collected is in the early morning, approximately 12 hours after the last ingestion of food.

3.

A. Since phlebotomy almost always causes some discomfort to the patient, this is not an accurate answer.

B. Basal state specimens are the most reliable. (p. 304)

C. Blood is not thicker during a basal state.

D. Most hospitals will schedule phlebotomists to work when it is most beneficial to the patient's health care. Blood collection during the basal state provides the most reliable results; thus, work shifts are often scheduled around this time of the morning. However, the work shifts are not usually preset prior to establishing high-quality laboratory practices.

4.

A. This is *not* standard procedure in all hospitals.

B. The specimen will *not* become diluted.

C. The patient may become dehydrated if he or she abstains from water for 12–24 hours. This can alter test results. It is important for the phlebotomist to explain the term fasting completely and ensure that the patient understands that they should abstain from food but not water. (p. 305)

D. The glucose level would not be elevated in this case.

5.

A.–D. (The correct answer is C.) More than half of adult patients in the United States are overweight. (p. 305)

6.

A. It is not appropriate for a patient to chew gum of any type prior to a "fasting glucose" procedure.

B. The phlebotomist should explain that chewing gum may cause a transient fluctuation in the blood sugar level. Furthermore, the phlebotomist could offer the patient a glass of water and ask the patient to please wait until after the procedure to chew gum. (p. 305)

C. The phlebotomist should *not* say it is okay to have coffee or tea.

D. The phlebotomist should *not* advise the patient to chew the gum for 5 minutes.

7.

A. The needle should be adjusted slightly to try to find the vein. Usually these patients know where the "best site" is for venipuncture, so it is helpful to check with the patient prior to the procedure. (p. 305)

B. Excessive probing is *not* recommended.

C. Pushing the needle all the way into the arm is *not* recommended.

D. The procedure should be discontinued only after trying to find the vein *without* excessive probing or discomfort to the patient.

8.

A. Excessive probing with a needle in the patient's arm can have a significant effect on a venipuncture specimen. It can cause rupturing of RBCs, increase the concentration of intracellular contents, and release some tissue-clotting factors.

B. Excessive probing with a needle in the patient's arm can have a significant effect on a venipuncture specimen. It can cause rupturing of RBCs, increase the concentration of intracellular contents, and release some tissue-clotting factors. (p. 305)

C. Excessive probing is *not* necessary and does not only alter the WBC count.

D. Excessive probing should *not* occur and thus, the physician would not be a factor.

9.

A.–D. (The correct answer is D.) Prolonged fasting and/or severe diets to lose weight can cause health hazards including electrolyte disturbances, cardiac dysrhythmias, and even death. (p. 305)

10.

A. An occluded vein is *not* larger than normal.

B. An occluded vein is *not* smaller than normal.

C. An occluded vein is obstructed and does not allow blood to flow through it. (p. 305)

D. An occluded vein does *not* usually refer to inflammation due to an infection.

11.

A.–D. (The correct answer is B.) If a patient is allergic to iodine and alcohol, chlorhexidine is an alternative to decontaminate the skin. It should be wiped off with sterile water after the application. (p. 306) The other answers are not appropriate.

12.

A.–D. (The correct answer is D.) The effects of exercise on laboratory tests are dependent on intensity, duration, frequency of the exercise,

and the individual's genetic factors, ethnicity, age, gender, hormonal status, and body weight. (p. 306)

13.

A. Edema does not refer to obesity.

B. Edema does not mean an infection of the skin.

C. Edema does not mean renal failure, although renal failure may cause edema.

D. Edema refers to an abnormal accumulation of fluid in the intercellular spaces. It may be caused after a mastectomy, or during heart or renal failure, bacterial toxins, or malnutrition. (p. 308)

14.

A. Excessive blood loss due to phlebotomy is *not* the most common cause of iron-deficiency anemia in women.

B. Hemorrhage is *not* the most common cause of iron-deficiency anemia in women.

C. Renal failure is *not* the most common cause of iron-deficiency anemia in women.

D. Menstrual blood loss is the most common cause of iron-deficiency anemia in women. Thus, it is vitally important that phlebotomists not withdraw more blood than is absolutely necessary so as not to increase the negative effects of additional blood loss during venipuncture. (p. 308)

15.

A and B. There is not a preset morning hour for collecting blood levels of medications.

C. This is not an appropriate answer.

D. In most cases, blood should be collected "just prior to the next dose" to determine blood levels of most medications. However, phlebotomists should realize that *each* medication has specific characteristics related to how the patient metabolizes the drug. Organizational policies/procedures should be carefully followed when collecting specimens for drug levels. (p. 308)

16.

A, B, C. Changing from a lying position to a sitting or standing position causes body water to shift from intravascular to interstitial compartments (in tissues), and certain larger molecules such as iron cannot filter into the tissue. Thus they concentrate in the blood. Testosterone, glucose, and cortisol are not significantly increased in the blood with changes in position.

D. Changing from a lying position to a sitting or standing position causes body water to shift from intravascular to interstitial compartments (in tissues), and certain larger molecules such as iron cannot filter into the tissue. Thus they concentrate in the blood. (p. 307)

17.

A. Lymphostasis means no lymph flow and occurs because of lymph node removal adjacent to the breast.

B. Thrombi are solid masses derived from blood constituents that reside in the blood vessels.

C. Thrombi are solid masses derived from blood constituents that reside in the blood vessels. (p. 310)

D. Petechiae are small red spots appearing on a patient's skin indicating that minute amounts of blood have escaped into skin epithelium.

18.

A.–D. (The correct answer is C.) If blood is to be collected for a timed blood glucose level determination, the patient needs to fast for 8 to 12 hours. Prolonged fasting has been shown to falsely alter blood test results. (p. 305)

19.

A. Cortisol is a hormone, and the blood concentration is not affected by light.

B. Bilirubin begins to deteriorate after 1 hour of exposure to light. (p. 319)

C. Testosterone is a hormone, and the blood concentration is not affected by light.

D. CPK is an enzyme and the blood concentration is not affected by light.

20.

A. Blood glucose levels are not significantly altered because of emotional stress or anxiety.

B. RBC counts are not significantly altered because of emotional stress or anxiety.

C. Emotional stress, such as anxiety or fear of blood collection, can lead to an increase in the WBC count. (p. 307)

D. Emotional stress, such as anxiety or fear of blood collection, can lead to a decrease in serum iron levels.

21.

A. Hyperventilation does not cause increased glucose levels.

B. Hyperventilation does not cause increased cell counts.

C. Hyperventilation does not cause increased serum iron.

D. Hyperventilation causes acid-base imbalances, increased lactate levels, and increased fatty acid levels. (p. 307)

22.

A,B,C. Aspirin should not have an altering effect on triglyceride or glucose levels, or red blood cell count.

D. Aspirin causes alterations in platelet functions, e.g., bleeding time. (pp. 309–310)

23.

A,B,D. A tourniquet should not be left on for more than 1 minute. The pressure of the tourniquet causes potassium to leak from the tissue cells into the blood, leading to falsely elevated values if the tourniquet pressure is prolonged.

C. The pressure of the tourniquet causes potassium to leak from the tissue cells into the blood, leading to falsely elevated values if the tourniquet pressure is prolonged. (p. 312)

24.

A, C, D. Basal state exists in the early morning, approximately 12 hours after the last ingestion of food.

B. Basal state exists in the early morning, approximately 12 hours after the last ingestion of food. (p. 304)

25.

A. An abnormal accumulation of fluid in the intercellular spaces of the body that is localized or diffused is referred to as edema. (p. 308)

B. Atherosclerosis is the accumulation of fat deposits within the blood vessels.

C. Hemolysis is the breakdown of red blood cells, releasing hemoglobin into the plasma.

D. Hemoconcentration refers to an increased concentration of larger molecules and formed elements in the blood.

26.

A. Atherosclerosis is the accumulation of fat deposits within the blood vessels.

B. Lymphostasis refers to no lymph flow.

C. When the area around the venipuncture site starts to swell, usually blood is leaking into the tissues and causing a hematoma. (p. 313)

D. Petechiae are small red spots appearing on a patient's skin and generally indicates that minute amounts of blood have escaped into skin epithelium.

27.

A. Diurnal rhythms are body fluid fluctuations during the day that affect certain blood analytes such as ACTH. (p. 307)

B, C, D. Diurnal rhythms are body fluid fluctuations during the day that affect certain blood analytes such as ACTH. They do not affect CK, cholesterol, or creatinine.

28.

A, B, D. The patient was lying on his back.

C. The term "supine" means that the patient was lying on his back. (p. 307)

29.

A. Fluorescein angiography can erroneously alter the blood creatinine, cortisol, and digoxin results. (p. 309)

B, C, D. Fluorescein angiography can erroneously alter the blood creatinine, cortisol, and digoxin results. It would not likely alter the reticulocyte count, RBC count, or WBC count.

30.

A. Growth hormone levels decrease with age.

B. Estrogen levels decrease in geriatric women.

C. Blood cholesterol and triglyceride levels increase with age. (p. 307)

D. Bilirubin levels are not affected by age alone.

31.

A. Another term for fainting is syncope. (p. 312)

B. Lymphostasis refers to no lymph flow and occurs due to lymph node removal.

C. Another term for fainting is syncope.

D. A thrombus is a solid mass derived from blood constituents that reside in blood vessels.

32.

A. "Falsely decreased" values of a blood analyte can be mistakenly interpreted as subnormal if the blood analyte is truly in an elevated range or a normal range. (pp. 309, 310)

B. Falsely decreased values of a blood analyte can be mistakenly interpreted as subnormal if the blood analyte is truly in an elevated range or a normal range.

C. Falsely decreased values of a blood analyte can be mistakenly interpreted as subnormal if the blood analyte is truly in an elevated range or a normal range.

D. All laboratory results are significant and important.

33.

A, B, C. A woman or man who has had a mastectomy (removal of a breast) may also have lymphostasis due to lymph node removal adjacent to the breast. Without lymph flow on that particular side of the body, the patient is highly susceptible to infection, and some blood analytes may be altered. Therefore, venipuncture should *not* be performed on the same side as that of a mastectomy. High blood pressure, cardiac bypass surgery, and heart attacks would not stop the phlebotomist from collecting blood from an arm vein.

D. A woman or man who has had a mastectomy (removal of a breast) may also have lymphostasis due to lymph node removal adjacent to the breast. Without lymph flow on that particular side of the body, the patient is highly susceptible to infection, and some blood analytes may be altered. Therefore, venipuncture should *not* be performed on the same side as that of a mastectomy. (p. 307)

34.

A, C, D. Smiling, syncope, and sneezing do not normally alter test results.

B. Violent crying can falsely alter laboratory test results dramatically. (p. 307)

35.

A, B, C. Anxiety that results in hyperventilation also causes acid-base imbalances, changing the blood pH level. It would not likely cause changes in triglyceride levels, RBC counts, or protein levels.

D. Anxiety that results in hyperventilation also causes acid-base imbalances, changing the blood pH level. (p. 307)

36.

A, B, C. Turbid serum appears cloudy or milky and can be a result of bacterial contamination or high lipid (i.e., cholesterol, triglyceride) levels in the blood.

D. Turbid serum appears cloudy or milky and can be a result of bacterial contamination or high lipid (i.e., cholesterol, triglyceride) levels in the blood. Elevated glucose results should not cause the serum to appear turbid. (p. 317)

37.

A. This woman's arm shows a hematoma close to the antecubital fossa area. A hematoma can occur when the needle has gone completely through a vein, the bevel opening is partially in the vein, or not enough pressure is applied to the site after puncture. (p. 315)

B, C, D. This woman's arm shows a hematoma close to the antecubital fossa area. A hematoma can occur when the needle has gone completely through a vein, the bevel opening is partially in the vein, or not enough pressure is applied to the site after puncture. It does not show lymphostasis, petechiae, or hemoconcentration.

38.

A. Hematomas are the result of a needle puncture that has gone completely through the vein, the bevel opening is partially in the vein, or not enough pressure is applied to the site after puncture.

B. Hemoconcentration is usually a complication of tourniquet application, massaging, squeezing, or probing a site.

C. Sclerosed, or hardened, veins are a result of inflammation and disease of the interstitial compartments after repeated venipunctures. (p. 305)

D. Syncope is another term for fainting, which occurs occasionally in patients who are having blood collections.

12 Pediatric Procedures

chapter objectives

Upon completion of Chapter 12, the learner is responsible for the following:

➤ Describe fears or concerns that children in different developmental stages might have toward the blood collection process.

➤ List suggestions that might be appropriate for parental behavior during a venipuncture or skin puncture.

➤ Identify puncture sites for a heel stick on an infant and describe the procedure.

➤ Describe the venipuncture sites for infants and young children.

➤ Discuss the types of equipment and supplies that must be used during microcollection and venipuncture of infants and children.

➤ Describe the procedure for specimen collection for neonatal phenylketonuria (PKU) and metabolic screening.

DIRECTIONS Each of the questions or incomplete statements below is followed by four suggested answers or completions. Select one answer that is best in each case.

1. EMLA is sometimes used for pediatric venipuncture procedures. EMLA is a:
   A. local anesthetic applied with a small needle to the child's arm before venipuncture
   B. topical anesthetic applied to the child's arm before venipuncture
   C. topical lotion applied to the child's arm after venipuncture to stop bleeding at the venipuncture site
   D. topical lotion applied to the child's arm before venipuncture to assist the phlebotomist in finding a vein

2. The best location for performing a phlebotomy on a hospitalized child is:
   A. at the bedside in a chair
   B. in a playroom
   C. in a treatment room
   D. in his or her bed

3. The optimal depth of a finger stick in a child is:
   A. greater than 3.0 mm
   B. less than 0.5 mm
   C. less than 3.0 mm
   D. less than 2.0 mm

4. What needle gauge is required for scalp vein venipuncture of an infant?
   A. 17
   B. 19
   C. 21
   D. 23

5. The angle of the needle for scalp vein venipuncture of an infant should be:
   A. 15 degrees
   B. 30 degrees
   C. 45 degrees
   D. 60 degrees

6. Complications resulting from multiple deep skin punctures on an infant's heel include:
   A. hepatitis
   B. AIDS
   C. pneumonia
   D. osteomyelitis

7. A commonly inherited disease that is detected through a blood screening process in neonates is:
   A. phenylketonuria
   B. spina bifida
   C. neurogenic bladder abnormality
   D. anemia

8. After a dorsal hand vein blood collection, pressure should be applied over the venipuncture site with a dry gauze sponge for:
   A. 20 to 30 seconds
   B. 30 to 60 seconds
   C. 1/2 to 1-1/2 minutes
   D. 2 to 3 minutes

9. The dorsal hand vein technique for infants includes which of the following steps?
   A. The patient's wrist veins are used.
   B. The health care provider collecting the sample uses a small Velcro-type tourniquet.

C. The infant is stuck with a safety lancet.

D. Blood is collected directly from the hub of a needle.

10. When a skin puncture is performed on an infant or a child, which of the following specimens is collected first?

A. blood bank specimens

B. chemistry specimens

C. clinical immunology specimens

D. hematology specimens

11. A 10-mL blood sample taken from a premature or newborn infant is equivalent to what percent of the infant's total blood volume?

A. 1 to 2 percent

B. 3 to 4 percent

C. 5 to 10 percent

D. 10 to 15 percent

12. Which of the following is needed for blood collection by skin puncture on an infant?

A. puncture-resistant sharps container

B. Eclipse safety needle

C. purple-topped evacuated tube

D. Velcro-type tourniquet

13. The total blood volume of a premature infant is calculated by multiplying weight in kilograms by:

A. 115 mL/kg

B. 80–110 mL/kg

C. 75–100 mL/kg

D. 70 mL/kg

14. Neonatal blood screening is required by law to test for:

A. hypoadrenalism

B. hypothyroidism

C. spina bifida

D. congenital neurogenic bladder anomaly

15. After the blood is collected from the newborn for PKU testing, the card must dry in a horizontal position for a minimum of:

A. 30 minutes

B. 1 hour

C. 2 hours

D. 4 hours

16. When collecting blood from a saline lock on a child, the blood collector must check the patency of the line by:

A. disinfecting the catheter cap with alcohol or povidone-iodine solution

B. flushing with a small amount of normal saline

C. injecting slowly the heparinized flush solution

D. flushing with a small amount of glucose solution

17. Which of the following is an acceptable intervention to alleviate pain during venipuncture on an infant or child?

A. xylocaine

B. sucrose nipple

C. ice pack

D. EMLA

18. Which is the preferred site for a heel stick?

A. anteromedial aspect

B. medial or lateral aspect

C. posterior curve

D. a previous puncture site

19. Compared with the skin puncture procedure, which of the following is true concerning the dorsal hand venipuncture procedure on an infant?
    A. It is more stressful for the infant.
    B. There is more dilution of the specimen with tissue fluid.
    C. Hemolysis occurs more often.
    D. Fewer punctures are required.

20. A premature infant weighing 2.0 kilograms has what total blood volume?
    A. 430 mL
    B. 230 mL
    C. 140 mL
    D. 160 mL

21. If 40 mL of blood is collected from a premature infant (weighing 4.0 kg) over a 2-day period, what percentage of the baby's total blood volume is that?
    A. 1%
    B. 2%
    C. 5%
    D. 10%

22. Figure 12.1 shows what vein to be used for blood collection from neonates and infants?
    A. median vein
    B. dorsal vein
    C. axillary vein
    D. cephalic vein

23. A latex-free tourniquet is absolutely necessary for a child with:
    A. chicken pox
    B. spina bifida
    C. congenital urinary tract abnormalities
    D. B and C are correct

FIGURE 12.1.

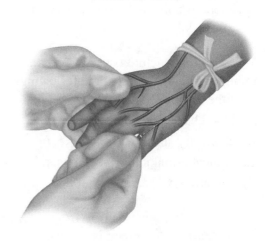

24. A child in what age group would perceive pain from a needlestick as a punishment for bad behavior?
    A. 1 year old
    B. 3 to 5 years old
    C. 6 to 10 years old
    D. 11 to 15 years old

25. Which is NOT a preferred sit for a heelstick?
    A. medial aspect
    B. lateral aspect
    C. central area
    D. lateral section of the plantar surface

26. In the collection of blood cultures from infants, which of the following is the preferred antiseptic to use prior to blood collection?
    A. 70% isopropyl alcohol
    B. chlorhexidine gluconate
    C. iodine
    D. Betadine

27. Venipuncture in children is indicated for which of the following laboratory tests?
    A. hemoglobin
    B. blood cultures
    C. WBC
    D. glucose

28. Which of the following is NOT a normal acceptable intervention to alleviate pain when performing venipuncture on an infant?
    A. EMLA cream
    B. oral sucrose
    C. lidocaine injection
    D. pacifier

29. When performing skin puncture on an infant or child, why are hematology specimens collected first?
    A. to minimize increased red blood cells in the microcollection containers
    B. to minimize platelet clumping
    C. to increase white and red blood cells in the containers for blood cell counts
    D. to maintain the proper blood pH

30. For a 3-year-old child, which of the following skin puncture sites is the most frequently used for blood collection?
    A. medial section of the bottom of the heel
    B. lateral section of the bottom of the heel
    C. palmar surface of the tip of the thumb
    D. palmar surface of the tip of the fourth finger

31. Blood spot testing for neonatal screening is performed before the newborn is:
    A. 24 hours old
    B. 36 hours old
    C. 48 hours old
    D. 72 hours old

32. Blood spot testing for neonatal screening to detect metabolic and genetic abnormalities occurs on blood collected from:
    A. the infant's scalp vein
    B. the median cubital vein
    C. the lateral plantar surface of the heel
    D. the dorsal vein

33. Figure 12.2 shows blood being collected for:
    A. blood gases
    B. hematology testing
    C. neonatal metabolic screening
    D. chemistry screening

34. To be effective, EMLA must be applied at least how long before venipuncture?
    A. 10 minutes
    B. 20 minutes
    C. 45 minutes
    D. 1 hour

35. What age group is embarrassed to show fear when venipuncture is performed on them?
    A. 1 to 3 years old
    B. 3 to 5 years old
    C. 6 to 12 years old
    D. 13 to 17 years old

FIGURE 12.2.

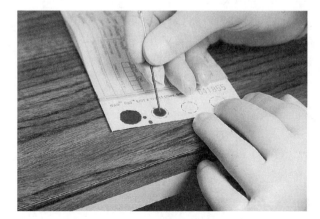

36. Isolation categories are based on the:
    A. vector
    B. mode of transmission
    C. genetic abnormality
    D. susceptible host

37. When performing skin punctures, the phlebotomist needs to collect chemistry specimens:
    A. first
    B. second
    C. third
    D. fourth

38. To collect blood from IV lines in a hospitalized child, which of the following is needed for a safe method to avoid a needlestick injury?
    A. transfer device for transferring blood to vacuum tubes
    B. butterfly needle for insertion into the IV line
    C. 21-gauge needle
    D. safety lancet

39. Why does OSHA mandate that latex or silicone membrane ports be used on CVCs?
    A. They are slippery and thus the needle can enter more easily into the port for blood collection.
    B. These ports can be easily disinfected before entry for blood collection.
    C. These ports allow penetration with a needless access device.
    D. Both B and C are correct.

40. When performing venipuncture on a child's arm, the recommended needle gauge is:
    A. 17
    B. 19

C. 21
D. 23

41. Newborns are routinely screened through blood analysis for which of the following genetic and metabolic defects?
    A. diabetes, congenital hypothyroidism
    B. PKU, galactosemia
    C. diabetes, PKU
    D. congenital hypothyroidism, obstructive jaundice

42. A sterile gauze sponge should be pressed against the infant's heel after skin puncture for blood collection in order to:
    A. avoid increased coagulation
    B. avoid a hematoma
    C. increase red blood cells to the site
    D. decrease calcium

43. What type of isolation category for a child warrants the use of a NIOSH-approved N-95 respirator?
    A. contact precautions
    B. droplet precautions
    C. airborne precautions
    D. direct precautions

44. A complication that can occur from a neonatal heelstick is:
    A. PKU
    B. congenital adrenal hyperplasia
    C. osteomyelitis
    D. toxoplasmosis

45. To prewarm the infant's heel for blood collection, it is best to prewarm the site for:
    A. 30 seconds
    B. 1 to 2 minutes

C. 3 to 5 minutes

D. 5 to 8 minutes

46. When collecting blood from a child's long-term CVC, what size syringe should be used?

A. 1 mL

B. 3 mL

C. 5 mL

D. 10 mL

47. Warming the infant's heel prior to blood collection provides which of the following benefits?

A. hastens hemostasis

B. increases blood flow

C. arterializes the blood specimen

D. both B and C are correct

48. For the performance of a heelstick on an infant, the infant should be positioned in the:

A. lateral position

B. supine position

C. prone position

D. recovery position

49. If a venipuncture needs to be performed on a child younger than 2 years of age, a recommended site is:

A. cephalic vein

B. axillary vein

C. medial wrist vein

D. basilic vein

50. In a child, the distance from the skin surface to bone or cartilage in the third finger is between:

A. 0.85 and 1.5 mm

B. 1.5 and 2.4 mm

C. 2.4 and 3.1 mm

D. 3.1 and 3.4 mm

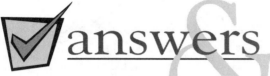

answers & rationales

1.

A, C, D. Eutectic mixture of local anesthetics (EMLA) is a topical anesthetic applied to the child's arm before venipuncture.

B. Eutectic mixture of local anesthetics (EMLA) is a topical anesthetic applied to the child's arm before venipuncture. (p. 336)

2.

A. For psychological reasons, the best room location for a painful procedure such as phlebotomy is not at the bedside.

B. For psychological reasons, the best room location for a painful procedure such as phlebotomy is not in a playroom.

C. For psychological reasons, the best room location for a painful procedure such as phlebotomy is a treatment room away from the child's bed or playroom. (p. 334)

D. For psychological reasons, the best room location for a painful procedure such as phlebotomy is not the child's bed or playroom.

3.

A, B, C. An automatic lancet should be used for the finger stick to a child, and the stick should not exceed 2.0 mm for small children.

D. An automatic lancet should be used for the finger stick to a child, and the stick should not exceed 2.0 mm for small children. (p. 340)

4.

A, B, C. A 17, 19, or 21 needle is not used for the venipuncture.

D. A 23- or 25-gauge safety winged infusion set (butterfly needle) is used for the venipuncture. (p. 351)

5.

A. Position the needle at a 15-degree angle over the infant's scalp vein in the direction of the blood flow. (p. 352)

B, C, D. Positioning the needle at a 30, 45, or 60 degree angle over the infant's scalp vein in the direction of the blood flow is not advisable.

6.

A. Hepatitis does not usually result from multiple deep skin punctures on an infant's heel.

B. AIDS does not usually result from multiple deep skin punctures on an infant's heel.

C. Pneumonia does not usually result from multiple deep skin punctures on an infant's heel.

D. Osteomyelitis can result from multiple deep skin punctures on an infant's heel. (p. 340)

7.

A. In the United States, neonatal blood screening for phenylketonuria (PKU) and hypothyroidism is mandatory by law. These diseases can result in severe abnormalities, including mental retardation. (p. 345)

B. Spina bifida is a congenital defect that is detected through a blood sample taken when the baby is still a fetus in the womb of the mother. Once the baby is born, the congenital abnormality is evident and not reversible.

C. In the United States, neonatal blood screening for phenylketonuria (PKU) and hypothyroidism is mandatory by law. These diseases can result in severe abnormalities, including mental retardation.

D. In the United States, neonatal blood screening for phenylketonuria (PKU) and hypothyroidism is mandatory by law. These diseases can result in severe abnormalities, including mental retardation.

8.

A, B, C. After the dorsal hand vein blood collection, pressure should be applied over the puncture site with a dry gauze sponge for 2 to 3 minutes.

D. After the dorsal hand vein blood collection, pressure should be applied over the puncture site with a dry gauze sponge for 2 to 3 minutes. (p. 350)

9.

A. The dorsal hand vein technique for neonates and infants does not require the use of wrist veins.

B. The dorsal hand vein technique for neonates and infants does not require the use of a tourniquet.

C. The dorsal hand vein technique for neonates and infants does not require the use of a safety lancet.

D. The dorsal hand vein technique for neonates and infants does not require the use of a tourniquet. The dorsal vein in the hand is used for the collection, and a needle is used to obtain the blood. The blood is collected directly from the hub of a needle. (p. 350)

10.

A, B, C. When a skin puncture is performed on an infant or a child, hematology specimens are collected first to minimize platelet clumping. Chemistry and blood bank specimens are collected next.

D. When a skin puncture is performed on an infant or a child, hematology specimens are collected first to minimize platelet clumping. (p. 339)

11.

A. A 10-mL blood sample taken from a premature or newborn infant is not equivalent to 1 to 2 percent of the infant's total blood volume.

B. A 10-mL blood sample taken from a premature or newborn infant is not equivalent to 3 to 4 percent of the infant's total blood volume.

C. A 10-mL blood sample taken from a premature or newborn infant is equivalent to 5 to 10 percent of the infant's total blood volume. (p. 338)

D. A 10-mL blood sample taken from a premature or newborn infant is not equivalent to 10 to 15 percent of the infant's total blood volume.

12.

A. For pediatric skin puncture, the following equipment is needed (p. 340):

1. **sterile automatic disposable pediatric safety lancet devices**
2. **70% isopropyl alcohol swabs in sterile packages**
3. **sterile cotton balls or gauze sponges**
4. **plastic capillary collection tubes and sealer**
5. **microcollection containers and Unopettes**
6. **glass slides for smears**
7. **puncture-resistant sharps container**
8. **disposable gloves (nonlatex if child is allergic)**
9. **compress (towel or washcloth) to warm heel, if necessary**
10. **marking pen**
11. **laboratory request slips or labels**

B, C, D. For pediatric skin puncture, the following equipment is needed:

1. sterile automatic disposable pediatric safety lancet devices
2. 70% isopropyl alcohol swabs in sterile packages
3. sterile cotton balls or gauze sponges
4. plastic capillary collection tubes and sealer
5. microcollection containers and Unopettes
6. glass slides for smears
7. puncture-resistant sharps container
8. disposable gloves (nonlatex if child is allergic)
9. compress (towel or washcloth) to warm heel, if necessary
10. marking pen
11. laboratory request slips or labels

13.

A. The total blood volume of a premature infant is calculated by multiplying the weight in kilograms by 115 mL/kg. (p. 338)

B. The total blood volume of a newborn infant is calculated by multiplying the baby's weight in kilograms by 80 to 110 mL/kg blood volume.

C. This is the blood volume calculation to be used for infants and children.

D. This is the blood volume calculation to be used for adults.

14.

A. In the United States, neonatal blood screening for hypoadrenalism is not mandatory by law.

B. In the United States, neonatal blood screening for phenylketonuria (PKU) and hypothyroidism is mandatory by law. (p. 345)

C. In the United States, neonatal blood screening for spina bifida is not mandatory by law.

D. In the United States, neonatal blood screening for congenital neurogenic bladder anomaly is not mandatory by law.

15.

A, B, C. After blood is collected for PKU testing, the card must thoroughly dry in a horizontal position for a minimum of 4 hours.

D. After blood is collected for PKU testing, the card must thoroughly dry in a horizontal position for a minimum of 4 hours. (p. 346)

16.

A. When collecting blood from a saline lock on a child, the blood collector must check the patency of the line by flushing with a small amount of normal saline.

B. When collecting blood from a saline lock on a child, the blood collector must check the patency of the line by flushing with a small amount of normal saline. (p. 354)

C. When collecting blood from a saline lock on a child, the blood collector must not check the patency of the line by injecting heparin.

D. When collecting blood from a saline lock on a child, the blood collector must not check the patency of the line by flushing with a small amount of glucose.

17.

A, B, C. The topical anesthetic EMLA (eutectic mixture of local anesthetics), which is an emulsion of lidocaine and prilocaine, can be applied to an infant or child to alleviate pain from venipuncture.

D. The topical anesthetic EMLA (eutectic mixture of local anesthetics), which is an emulsion of lidocaine and prilocaine, can be applied to an infant or child to alleviate pain from venipuncture. (p. 336)

18.

A. The anteromedial aspect or the posterior curve of the heel must not be used for a skin puncture site because a puncture at either site could injure the underlying calcaneus.

B. The preferred site for a heel stick is the medial or lateral aspect of the heel. (p. 339)

C. The anteromedial aspect or the posterior curve of the heel must not be used for a skin puncture site because a puncture at either site could injure the underlying calcaneus.

D. Avoid heel sticks in an area that has previous puncture sites because such a stick could cause an infection.

19.

A, B, D. Compared with skin puncture, dorsal hand venipuncture on an infant is less stressful for the infant and the health care provider, there is less dilution of the specimen with tissue fluids, there is less hemolysis, and fewer punctures are required.

C. Compared with skin puncture, dorsal hand venipuncture on an infant is less stressful for the infant and the health care provider, there is less dilution of the specimen with tissue fluids, there is less hemolysis, and fewer punctures are required. (p. 351)

20.

A. A premature infant weighing 2.0 kg will not have a total blood volume of 430 mL.

B. A premature infant weighing 2.0 kg will have a total blood volume of 115 mL/kg $\times$ 2 kg = 230 mL. (p. 338)

C. A premature infant weighing 2.0 kg will probably have a total blood volume of greater than 140 mL.

D. A premature infant weighing 2.0 kg will probably have a total blood volume of greater than 160 mL.

21.

A. If 40 mL of blood is collected from a newborn infant (weighing 4.0 kg) over a 3-day period, that is greater than 1% of the infant's total blood volume.

B. If 40 mL of blood is collected from a newborn infant (weighing 4.0 kg) over a 3-day period, that is greater than 2% of the infant's total blood volume.

C. If 40 mL of blood is collected from a newborn infant (weighing 4.0 kg) over a 3-day period, that is greater than 5% of the infant's total blood volume.

D. If 40 mL of blood is collected from a newborn infant (weighing 4.0 kg) over a 3-day period, that is equivalent to approximately 10% of the infant's total blood volume. (p. 338)

22.

A. Figure 12.1 does not show the median vein.

B. Figure 12.1 shows the dorsal hand vein that is appropriate for blood collection from neonates and infants. (p. 349)

C. Figure 12.1 does not show the axillary vein.

D. Figure 12.1 does not show the cephalic vein.

23.

A, B, C. Children with spina bifida and those with congenital urinary tract abnormalities are particularly sensitive to latex and thus a tourniquet that is latex-free should be used when collecting their blood.

D. Children with spina bifida and those with congenital urinary tract abnormalities are particularly sensitive to latex and thus a tourniquet that is latex-free should be used when collecting their blood. (p. 338)

24.

A, C, D. Children 3 to 5 years old perceive pain as a punishment for bad behavior and will most likely perceive a needlestick as punishment for bad behavior.

FIGURE 12.1. Hand veins.

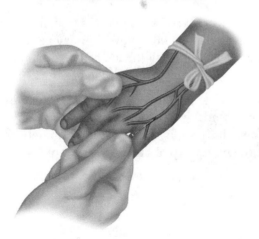

B. Children 3 to 5 years old perceive pain as a punishment for bad behavior and will most likely perceive a needlestick as punishment for bad behavior. (p. 334)

25.

A. The medial or most lateral section of the plantar surface of the heel should be used.

B. The medial or most lateral section of the plantar surface of the heel should be used.

C. The medial or most lateral section of the plantar surface of the heel should be used, NOT the central area. (p. 339)

D. The medial or most lateral section of the plantar surface of the heel should be used.

26.

A. For blood culture collections from an infant, 70% isopropyl alcohol is not the preferred antiseptic.

B. For blood culture collections from an infant, chlorhexidine gluconate swabs should be used rather than iodine for their sensitive skin. (p. 349)

C. For blood culture collections from an infant, iodine is not the preferred antiseptic.

D. For blood culture collections from an infant, Betadine is not the preferred antiseptic.

27.

A. Hemoglobin testing can occur on blood collected by skin puncture on a child.

B. Blood cultures require large amounts of blood that must be collected by venipuncture. (p. 348)

C. WBC (white blood cell) count can occur on blood collected by skin puncture on a child.

D. Glucose results can be obtained from a blood sample collected by skin puncture on a child.

28.

A, B, D. EMLA cream, oral sucrose, a pacifier, and swaddling are the normal acceptable methods to alleviate pain from venipuncture in an infant.

C. EMLA cream, oral sucrose, a pacifier and swaddling are the normal acceptable methods to alleviate pain from venipuncture in an infant. (pp. 336–337)

29.

A. When performing skin puncture on infants or children, the phlebotomist does not collect the hematology specimens first to minimize increased red blood cells.

B. When performing skin puncture on infants or children, the phlebotomist collects the hematology specimens first to minimize platelet clumping. (p. 339)

C. When performing skin puncture on infants or children, the phlebotomist does not collect the hematology specimens first to increase WBCs and RBCs.

D. When performing skin puncture on infants or children, the phlebotomist does not collect the hematology specimens first to maintain proper blood pH.

30.

A, B. For children older than 1 year, the heelstick is not preferred.

C. For children older than 1 year, the palmar surface of the tip of the third or fourth finger is most frequently used.

D. For children older than 1 year, the palmar surface of the tip of the third or fourth finger is most frequently used. (p. 339)

31.

A, B, C. Blood spot testing for neonatal screening is performed before the newborn is 72 hours old.

D. Blood spot testing for neonatal screening is performed before the newborn is 72 hours old. (p. 345)

32.

A. Blood collection for neonatal screening to detect metabolic and genetic defects does not occur on the infant's scalp vein.

B. Blood collection for neonatal screening to detect metabolic and genetic defects does not occur on the median cubital vein.

C. Blood collection for neonatal screening to detect metabolic and genetic defects occurs on the lateral or medial plantar surface of the heel. (p. 346)

D. Blood collection for neonatal screening to detect metabolic and genetic defects occurs on the lateral or medial plantar surface of the heel.

33.

A. Figure 12.2 does not show blood being collected for blood gases.

B. Figure 12.2 does not show blood being collected for hematology testing.

C. Figure 12.2 shows blood being collected for neonatal metabolic screening. (p. 347)

D. Figure 12.2 shows blood being collected for neonatal metabolic screening.

FIGURE 12.2. Collecting a blood sample from the newborn for neonatal metabolic screening.

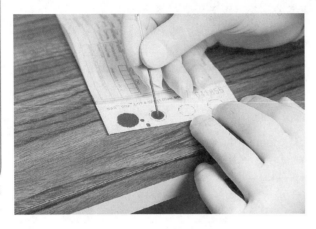

34.

A. For optimal effectiveness, EMLA should be applied longer than 10 minutes before venipuncture.

B. For optimal effectiveness, EMLA should be applied longer than 20 minutes before venipuncture.

C. For optimal effectiveness, EMLA should be applied longer than 45 minutes before venipuncture.

D. For optimal effectiveness, EMLA should be applied at least 1 hour before venipuncture. (p. 336)

35.

A, B, C. The age group of 13 to 17 years old is embarrassed to show fear during venipuncture.

D. The age group of 13 to 17 years old is embarrassed to show fear during venipuncture. (pp. 330–331)

36.

A. Isolation categories are not based on the vector.

B. Isolation categories are based on the mode of transmission. (p. 337)

C. Isolation categories are not based on genetic abnormality.

D. Isolation categories are not based on the susceptible host.

37.

A, C, D. When performing skin punctures, the phlebotomist collects the hematology specimens first, then the chemistry specimens with additives are second.

B. When performing skin punctures, the phlebotomist collects the hematology specimens first, then the chemistry specimens with additives are second. (pp. 339, 295)

38.

A. To collect blood from an IV line in a child, a syringe that can enter a needleless cannula is the safe method to enter into the line for blood collection. Thus, after collection, a transfer device is needed to transfer the blood to the vacuum tubes. (pp. 352–354)

B, C, D. To collect blood from an IV line in a child, a syringe that can enter a needleless cannula is the safe method to enter into the line for blood collection. Thus, after collection, a transfer device is needed to transfer the blood to the vacuum tubes.

39.

A, B, C. OSHA mandates that latex or silicone membrane ports be used on CVCs because the ports allow penetration with a needleless access device and can easily be disinfected before entry.

D. OSHA mandates that latex or silicone membrane ports be used on CVCs because the ports allow penetration with a needleless ac-

cess device and can easily be disinfected before entry. (p. 352)

40.

A, B, C. When performing venipuncture on a child's arm, it is recommended to use a winged safety infusion needle that is 23- or 25-gauge.

D. When performing venipuncture on a child's arm, it is recommended to use a winged safety infusion needle that is 23- or 25-gauge. (p. 349)

41.

A. Newborns are routinely screened through blood analysis for a variety of metabolic and genetic defects that include congenital hypothyroidism, but not diabetes.

B. Newborns are routinely screened through blood analysis for a variety of metabolic and genetic defects that include PKU, congenital hypothyroidism, galactosemia, homocystinuria, congenital adrenal hyperplasia, and sickle cell disease. (p. 345)

C. Newborns are routinely screened through blood analysis for a variety of metabolic and genetic defects that include PKU, but not diabetes.

D. Newborns are routinely screened through blood analysis for a variety of metabolic and genetic defects that include congenital hypothyroidism, but not obstructive jaundice.

42.

A, C, D. The infant's heel should have a sterile gauze pressed against the skin puncture site after blood collection to avoid the formation of a hematoma.

B. The infant's heel should have a sterile gauze pressed against the skin puncture site after blood collection to avoid the formation of a hematoma. (p. 344)

43.

A, B, D. Isolation categories are based on the mode of transmission: contact, droplet, or airborne. If a child is on airborne precautions, a NIOSH-approved N-95 respirator must be used.

C. Isolation categories are based on the mode of transmission: contact, droplet, or airborne. If a child is on airborne precautions, a NIOSH-approved N-95 respirator must be used. (p. 337)

44.

A. Some complications that can occur due to neonatal heel sticks does not include PKU.

B. Some complications that can occur due to neonatal heel sticks does not include congenital adrenal hyperplasia.

C. Some complications that can occur due to neonatal heel sticks include: celluitis, osteomyelitis, and scarring of the heel. (p. 344)

D. Some complications that can occur due to neonatal heel sticks does not include toxoplasmosis.

45.

A, B, D. The infant's heel should be prewarmed for 3 to 5 minutes prior to the heel stick.

C. The infant's heel should be prewarmed for 3 to 5 minutes prior to the heel stick. (p. 344)

46.

A. When collecting blood from a child's long-term CVC, a 1 mL syringe is too small.

B. When collecting blood from a child's long-term CVC, a 3 mL syringe is too small.

C. When collecting blood from a child's long-term CVC, a 5 mL syringe is too small.

D. When collecting blood from a child's long-term CVC, use a 10 mL or larger syringe to avoid overpressurizing and rupture of the catheter. (p. 352)

47.

A, B, C. Prewarming the infant's heel prior to blood collection increases the blood flow and arterializes the blood specimen.

D. Prewarming the infant's heel prior to blood collection increases the blood flow and arterializes the blood specimen. (p. 344)

48.

A, C, D. When performing a heel stick on an infant, position the infant in the supine position (face up).

B. When performing a heel stick on an infant, position the infant in the supine position (face up). (p. 341)

49.

A, B, D. If a venipuncture is needed for larger amounts of blood on a child younger than 2 years of age, the medial wrist and the scalp are two acceptable sites for the venipuncture.

C. If a venipuncture is needed for larger amounts of blood on a child younger than 2 years of age, the medial wrist and the scalp are two acceptable sites for the venipuncture. (p. 346)

50.

A, C, D. In a child, the distance from the skin surface to bone or cartilage in the third finger is between 1.5 and 2.4 mm. Thus, an automatic skin-puncture device should not exceed 2.0 mm in small children.

B. In a child, the distance from the skin surface to bone or cartilage in the third finger is between 1.5 and 2.4 mm. Thus, an automatic skin-puncture device should not exceed 2.0 mm in small children. (p. 346)

13 Arterial, Intravenous (IV), and Special Collection Procedures

chapter objectives

Upon completion of Chapter 13, the learner is responsible for the following:

➤ Explain the special precautions and types of equipment needed to collect capillary or arterial blood gases.

➤ Describe the equipment that is used to perform the bleeding-time test.

➤ Discuss the requirements for the glucose and lactose tolerance tests.

➤ Differentiate cannulas from fistulas.

➤ List the steps and equipment in blood culture collections.

➤ List the special requirements for collecting blood through intravenous (IV) catheters.

➤ Differentiate therapeutic phlebotomy from autologous transfusion.

➤ Describe the special precautions needed to collect blood in therapeutic drug monitoring (TDM) procedures.

➤ List the types of patient specimens that are needed for trace metal analyses.

DIRECTIONS Each of the questions or incomplete statements below is followed by four suggested answers or completions. Select one answer that is best in each case.

1. Cleansing the venipuncture site before collection of blood culture specimens usually involves the use of:
   A. isopropyl alcohol and peroxide
   B. ethyl alcohol and peroxide
   C. iodine and peroxide
   D. iodine and alcohol

2. Which of the following is the specimen of choice for testing the pH, pO_2, and pCO_2 of the blood?
   A. arterial blood
   B. venous blood
   C. heparinized plasma
   D. skin puncture blood

3. Which of the following sites is *not* recommended to collect capillary blood gases?
   A. lateral posterior area of the heel
   B. lateral anterior area of the elbow
   C. medial plantar area of the heel
   D. the ball of the finger

4. What anticoagulant should be used to collect a specimen for capillary blood gas analysis?
   A. heparin
   B. EDTA
   C. lidocaine
   D. sodium citrate

5. Which of the following supplies is *not* needed during an arterial puncture for an ABG determination?
   A. syringe
   B. tourniquet

C. gloves
D. lidocaine

6. When blood is collected from the radial artery for an arterial blood gas collection, the needle should be inserted at an angle of no less than:
   A. 15 degrees
   B. 25 degrees
   C. 35 degrees
   D. 45 degrees

7. Which of the following is the preferred site for blood collection for arterial blood gas analysis?
   A. ulnar artery
   B. femoral artery
   C. radial artery
   D. subclavian artery

8. What is the rationale for performing the Allen test?
   A. To test for the possibility of edema.
   B. To determine whether the patient's blood pressure is elevated.
   C. To determine that the radial and ulnar arteries are providing collateral circulation.
   D. To determine whether the oxygen concentration in the radial artery is sufficient for blood collection.

9. Which of the following evacuated tubes is preferred for the collection of arterial blood gas analysis?
   A. yellow-topped evacuated tube
   B. green-topped evacuated tube

C. light blue–topped evacuated tube

D. no evacuated tube

10. Which of the following evacuated tubes is preferred for the collection of a blood culture specimen?

A. yellow-topped evacuated tube

B. green-topped evacuated tube

C. speckled-topped evacuated tube

D. light blue–topped evacuated tube

11. What is a cannula?

A. a good source of arterial blood

B. the fusion of a vein and an artery

C. a tubular instrument used to gain access to venous blood

D. an artificial shunt that provides access to arterial blood

12. For central venous catheter (CVC) blood collections, which of the following blood analytes has to have 7 mL of blood discarded from the line before another separate syringe is used to collect an additional amount for the analyte test?

A. CPK

B. PT

C. ALT

D. AST

13. The bleeding-time test is used to:

A. check for vascular abnormalities

B. diagnose diabetes mellitus

C. determine whether the patient's blood pressure is low

D. access liver glycogen stores

14. Which of the following tubes must be collected first?

A. red-topped evacuated tube

B. yellow-topped evacuated tube

C. light blue–topped evacuated tube

D. royal blue–topped evacuated tube

15. Which of the following is used to help in the diagnosis of diabetes mellitus?

A. ABG analysis

B. PT

C. TDM

D. GTT

16. *Postprandial* refers to:

A. 2-hour fasting

B. 12-hour fasting

C. after eating

D. before eating

17. Which of the following is the appropriate volume of blood to collect from a blood donor?

A. 450 mL

B. 150 mL

C. 100 mL

D. 50 mL

18. Resin beads to neutralize antibiotics in the blood specimen are used in the:

A. heparin lock system for IV blood collections

B. bleeding-time test

C. blood culture collections

D. special arterial blood gas collections

19. To obtain the blood trough level for a medication, the patient's blood should be collected:

A. immediately after administration of the medication

B. immediately before administration of the medication

C. 2 hours before administration of the medication

D. 2 hours after administration of the medication

20. Which of the following tests requires numerous blood collections?
    A. arterial blood gas analysis
    B. GTT
    C. bleeding-time test
    D. drug screening

21. Which of the following procedures requires blood collection for trough- and peak-level determinations?
    A. skin test for allergies
    B. therapeutic drug monitoring
    C. blood collection through CVCs
    D. sweat chloride procedure

22. Which of the following procedures helps to reduce potential scarring from the Surgicutt bleeding-time test?
    A. Apply a butterfly-type bandage to the incision site.
    B. Provide a small stitch to the incision site.
    C. Apply gauze and tape to the incision site.
    D. Apply a small piece of moleskin to the incision site.

23. For the Surgicutt bleeding-time test, the blood pressure cuff must be inflated on the patient's upper arm to
    A. 20 mm Hg
    B. 30 mm Hg
    C. 40 mm Hg
    D. 60 mm Hg

24. The health care worker's thumb should not be used for palpating arteries in the arterial puncture procedure because the thumb:
    A. is usually dirty
    B. has less sensitivity than the other fingers
    C. has a pulse that may be confused with the patient's pulse

D. has more neurons for touching, which interfere in the process of finding the patient's pulse

25. Blood gas analyses include testing for:
    A. pH, pH_2O, and pCO_2
    B. pH, pO_2, and pCO_2
    C. pH_2O, pCO_2, and pO_2
    D. pH_2O, pH, and pO_2

26. If the patient's bleeding time is longer than the normal limits, which of the following laboratory tests may be needed?
    A. alkaline phosphatase level
    B. acid phosphatase level
    C. platelet count
    D. blood urea nitrogen result

27. Which of the following procedures requires a syrine with needleless cannula containing 10 mL of heparinized saline and a 10-mL disposable syringe with needleless cannula?
    A. sweat chloride procedure
    B. skin test for allergies
    C. blood collection from a blood donor
    D. blood collection through CVCs

28. Which of the following is frequently used as a preoperative screening test?
    A. GTT
    B. bleeding-time test
    C. blood cultures
    D. lactose tolerance test

29. Which of the following guidelines must the patient abide by to properly prepare him- or herself for the GTT?
    A. The patient's carbohydrate intake must not exceed 20 g per day for 3 days before the GTT.

B. The patient must not eat anything for 12 hours before the GTT but should not fast for more than 14 hours before the test.

C. The patient should take corticosteroids 2 days before the GTT

D. The patient should vigorously exercise within 8 to 12 hours before the GTT.

30. Which of the following drugs has a shorter half-life and therefore requires exact timing in blood collection for its therapeutic level?

A. procainamide

B. phenobarbital

C. digoxin

D. digitoxin

31. Normally, after an adult patient ingests the 75 or 100 g of glucose in the glucose tolerance test, the glucose level should return to normal within how many minutes?

A. 30

B. 60

C. 120

D. 180

32. Before a blood donation, the phlebotomist must always check the blood donor's:

A. blood glucose value

B. hematocrit or hemoglobin value

C. urine glucose value

D. WBC count

33. An autologous transfusion is used to prevent which of the following possibilities?

A. Polycythemia will develop in the transfused patient.

B. Antigens will form in the transfused patient.

C. Antibodies will form in the transfused patient.

D. The transfused patient will develop diabetes mellitus.

34. During a glucose tolerance test, which procedure is acceptable?

A. A standard amount of glucose drink is given to the patient, then a fasting blood collection is performed.

B. The patient should be encouraged to drink water throughout the procedure.

C. The patient is allowed to chew sugarless gum.

D. All the patient's specimens are timed from the fasting collection.

35. Which of the following is a milk sugar that sometimes cannot be digested by healthy individuals?

A. glucose

B. glucagon

C. lactose

D. lactate

36. Which of the following is the correct protocol in the collection of blood for blood cultures?

A. palpating the venipuncture site after the site has been prepared without first cleaning the chemically cleaned gloved finger

B. injecting air into the anaerobic bottle

C. inoculating the anaerobic bottle last

D. wiping the iodine from the tops of the bottles with alcohol

37. The following materials and/or supplies are needed for the Surgicutt procedure except:

A. blood pressure cuff

B. butterfly-type bandage

C. disposable gloves

D. vacuum blood collection tube with EDTA

38. Figure 13.1 shows swabbing of the arm in concentric circles in preparation of collecting blood for:
    A. therapeutic drug monitoring
    B. toxicology studies
    C. blood donation
    D. lactose tolerance test

39. A tubular instrument that is used in kidney patients to gain access to venous blood for dialysis or blood collection is referred to as a:
    A. CVC
    B. cannula
    C. fistula
    D. Venous isolator

40. Therapeutic phlebotomy is used in the treatment of:
    A. megaloblastic anemia
    B. polycythemia
    C. chronic anemia
    D. iron-deficiency anemia

41. To help minimize the incidence of dizziness, fainting, or other reactions to blood loss, blood donors are encouraged to eat within how many hours of donating blood?
    A. 9
    B. 8
    C. 7
    D. 6

42. Which of the following items is *not* usually kept on file for every blood donor indefinitely?
    A. age
    B. a written consent form signed by the donor
    C. a record of reason for deferrals
    D. a written consent form signed by the donor's parent

43. For a donor to donate blood, his or her oral temperature must not exceed:
    A. 35°C
    B. 37.5°C
    C. 38.7°C
    D. 39.5°F

44. For the brief physical examination that is required to determine whether a blood donor is in generally good health, the donor's systolic blood pressure should measure no higher than:
    A. 100 mm Hg
    B. 110 mm Hg
    C. 180 mm Hg
    D. 190 mm Hg

FIGURE 13.1.

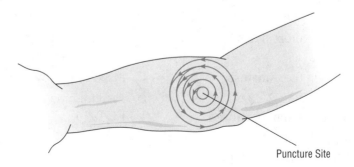

Puncture Site

45. A false-negative blood culture is more likely to occur if:
    A. iodine is not wiped from the tops of the blood culture tubes
    B. the indwelling catheter is used to obtain the culture specimen
    C. too much blood is used for the culture
    D. the health care worker palpates the venipuncture site after the site has been prepared without first cleaning the gloved finger

46. Blood glucose levels are measured for patients undergoing:
    A. Allen test
    B. blood gas analysis
    C. lactose tolerance test
    D. therapeutic phlebotomy

47. Which of the following can lead to deferral of a person from blood donation?
    A. weighs 110 pounds
    B. has an oral temperature of 37°C
    C. has a hematocrit value of 36%
    D. has a pulse rate of 70 beats per minute

48. Which of the following can lead to deferral of a person from blood donation? The potential donor has:
    A. a poison ivy rash on his or her arms
    B. purulent skin lesions on his or her arms
    C. psoriasis skin lesions on his or her arms
    D. acne skin lesions on his or her arms

49. If a potential donor is allergic to iodine, then in venipuncture site preparation for blood donation, the phlebotomist should use which of the following?
    A. 1% PVP without iodine
    B. alcohol only
    C. soap/acetone alcohol
    D. 0.75% PVP-iodine

50. An artificial shunt in which the vein and artery have been fused through surgery is usually found in:
    A. cardiac patients
    B. kidney dialysis patients
    C. patients with liver disease
    D. patients with arm amputations

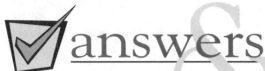

answers & rationales

1.

A. Cleansing the venipuncture site before collection of blood culture specimens does not usually involve the use of isopropyl alcohol and peroxide.

B. Cleansing the venipuncture site before collection of blood culture specimens does not usually involve the use of ethyl alcohol and peroxide.

C. Cleansing the venipuncture site before collection of blood culture specimens does not usually involve the use of iodine and peroxide.

D. Cleansing the venipuncture site before collection of blood culture specimens usually involves the use of iodine and alcohol. (pp. 372–373)

2.

A. Arterial blood is the specimen of choice for testing the pH, pO$_2$, and pCO$_2$ of the blood. Arterial blood is used rather than venous blood because arterial blood has the same composition throughout the body tissues, whereas venous blood has various compositions relative to metabolic activities in body tissues. (p. 362)

B, C, D. Arterial blood is the specimen of choice for testing the pH, pO$_2$, and pCO$_2$ of the blood. Arterial blood is used rather than venous blood because arterial blood has the same composition throughout the body tissues, whereas venous blood has various compositions relative to metabolic activities in body tissues.

3.

A, C, D. Blood for capillary blood gas analysis is collected from the same areas of the body as other capillary samples, such as the lateral posterior area of the heel or the ball of the finger.

B. Blood for capillary blood gas analysis is collected from the same areas of the body as other capillary samples, such as the lateral posterior area of the heel or the ball of the finger. (p. 367)

4.

A. A heparinized capillary tube with a volume of at least 100 μL should be used to collect a specimen for capillary blood gas analysis. (p. 368)

B. EDTA should not be used to collect for capillary blood gas analysis.

C. Lidocaine should not be used to collect for capillary blood gas analysis.

D. Sodium citrate should not be used to collect for capillary blood gas analysis.

5.

A. As in venipuncture, a syringe with a needle is used to collect the blood.

B. No tourniquet is required because the artery has its own strong blood pressure. (pp. 362–366)

C. As in any blood collection procedure, gloves are required for the procedure.

D. Lidocaine, in ½ to 1%, is needed to numb the site.

6.

A. The health care worker should pierce the pulsating artery at a high angle, not 15 degrees.

B. The health care worker should pierce the pulsating artery at a high angle, not 25 degrees.

C. The health care worker should pierce the pulsating artery at a high angle, not 35 degrees.

D. The health care worker should pierce the pulsating artery at a high angle, usually no less than 45 degrees. (p. 367)

7.

A, B, D. When an arterial blood gas analysis is ordered, the health care worker should palpate the radial artery in the radial sulcus of the forearm, since the radial artery in the patient's nondominant hand is usually the best choice.

C. When an arterial blood gas analysis is ordered, the health care worker should palpate the radial artery in the radial sulcus of the forearm, since the radial artery in the patient's nondominant hand is usually the best choice. (p. 362)

8.

A. To use the radial artery for blood collection for arterial blood gas analysis, the health care provider does not test for edema.

B. To use the radial artery for blood collection for arterial blood gas analysis, the health care provider does not first check blood pressure.

C. To use the radial artery for blood collection for arterial blood gas analysis, the health care provider must first perform the Allen test to make certain that the ulnar and radial arteries are providing collateral circulation. (p. 363)

D. To use the radial artery for blood collection for arterial blood gas analysis, the health care provider must first perform the Allen test to make certain that the ulnar and radial arteries are providing collateral circulation.

9.

A, B, C. For the radial artery blood gas collection, a safety syringe is used, since little or no suction is needed because the blood pulsates and flows quickly into the syringe under its own pressure.

D. For the radial artery blood gas collection, a safety syringe is used, since little or no suction is needed because the blood pulsates and flows quickly into the syringe under its own pressure. (p. 367)

10.

A. Blood culture specimens need to be collected in SPS (yellow-topped) evacuated tubes. (pp. 372, 375)

B. Blood culture specimens are not collected in green-topped evacuated tubes.

C. Blood culture specimens are not collected in specked-topped evacuated tubes.

D. Blood culture specimens are not collected in light blue-topped evacuated tubes.

11.

A. A cannula is not a good source of arterial blood.

B and D. A cannula is a tubular instrument that is used in patients with kidney disease to gain access to venous blood for dialysis or blood collections.

C. A cannula is a tubular instrument that is used in patients with kidney disease to gain access to venous blood for dialysis or blood collections. (p. 385)

12.

A. The CPK test does not have to have blood aspirated with a syringe from the line and discarded before 3 mL is aspirated from the line with another syringe that is then used for the blood analysis.

B. The coagulation tests, protime (PT) and partial thromboplastin time (PTT), have to have 7 mL of blood discarded before 3 mL is aspirated from the line with another syringe that is then used for the blood analysis. (p. 386)

C. The ALT analysis does not have to have blood aspirated with a syringe from the line and discarded before 3 mL is aspirated from the line with another syringe that is then used for the blood analysis.

D. The AST analysis does not have to have blood aspirated with a syringe from the line and discarded before 3 mL is aspirated from the line with another syringe that is then used for the blood analysis.

13.

A. The bleeding-time test is a useful tool for testing platelet plug formation in the capillaries to diagnose coagulopathies or problems in hemostasis, such as vascular abnormalities. (p. 368)

B. The bleeding-time test is not a useful tool for testing for diabetes mellitus.

C. The bleeding-time test is not a useful tool for testing blood pressure.

D. The bleeding-time test is not a useful tool for testing glycogen stores.

14.

A, C, D. If blood culture collections are ordered with other laboratory tests, blood culture specimens (i.e., collected in the SPS yellow-topped evacuated tube) must be collected first to avoid contamination of the blood specimen.

B. If blood culture collections are ordered with other laboratory tests, blood culture specimens (i.e., collected in the SPS yellow-topped evacuated tube) must be collected first to avoid contamination of the blood specimen. (p. 375)

15.

A. The arterial blood gas (ABG) analysis is used to detect respiratory and acid-base imbalances in patients.

B. The protime (PT) is a coagulation test used to detect abnormal clotting in patients.

C. Therapeutic drug monitoring (TDM) is used to monitor the serum concentration of certain drugs such as anticonvulsant drugs, tricyclic antidepressants, and digoxin.

D. The glucose tolerance test (GTT) can be an effective diagnostic tool for patients who have symptoms suggesting problems in carbohydrate metabolism. (p. 376)

16.

A, B, D. *Postprandial* means "after eating."

C. *Postprandial* means "after eating." (p. 380)

17.

A. The appropriate volume of blood to collect from a blood donor is 450 mL. (p. 484)

B, C, D. The appropriate volume of blood to collect from a blood donor is 450 mL.

18.

A. Resin beads that neutralize antibiotics in the patient's blood specimen are not used in the heparin lock system.

B. Resin beads that neutralize antibiotics in the patient's blood specimen are not used in the bleeding time test.

C. Resin beads that neutralize antibiotics in the patient's blood specimen are used in the blood culture collections. (p. 376)

D. Resin beads that neutralize antibiotics in the patient's blood specimen are not used in the blood gas collections.

19.

A, C, D. To obtain the blood trough level for a medication, the patient's blood should be collected immediately before the administration of the medication. The trough level is the lowest concentration in the patient's serum.

B. To obtain the blood trough level for a medication, the patient's blood should be collected immediately before the administration of the medication. The trough level is the lowest concentration in the patient's serum. (pp. 381–382)

20.

A. The arterial blood gas analysis requires only one arterial blood collection.

B. The glucose tolerance test (GTT) is performed by obtaining fasting blood and urine specimens, giving the fasting patient a stan-dard load of glucose, and obtaining subsequent blood and urine specimens at intervals, usually during a 5-hour period. (p. 377)

C. The bleeding-time test requires only one blood collection.

D. Drug screening usually requires a urine specimen or one blood collection.

21.

A, C, D. So that physicians can adequately evaluate the appropriate dosage levels of many drugs, the collection and evaluation of specimens for trough and peak levels are necessary in therapeutic drug monitoring.

B. So that physicians can adequately evaluate the appropriate dosage levels of many drugs, the collection and evaluation of specimens for trough and peak levels are necessary in therapeutic drug monitoring. (pp. 381–382)

22.

A. Applying a butterfly-type bandage to the incision area for a 24-hour period can reduce the scarring that may result from a Surgicutt bleeding-time test. (p. 370)

B, C, D. Applying a butterfly-type bandage to the incision area for a 24-hour period can reduce the scarring that may result from a Surgicutt bleeding-time test.

23.

A, B, D. For the Surgicutt bleeding-time test, the blood pressure cuff must be inflated on the patient's upper arm to 40 mm Hg.

C. For the Surgicutt bleeding-time test, the blood pressure cuff must be inflated on the patient's upper arm to 40 mm Hg. (p. 370)

24.

A, B, D. The health care provider's thumb should not be used for palpating arteries in the arterial puncture procedure because the thumb has a pulse that may be confused with the patient's pulse.

C. The health care provider's thumb should not be used for palpating arteries in the arterial puncture procedure because the thumb has a pulse that may be confused with the patient's pulse. (p. 367)

25.

A. Blood gas analyses do not include testing for pH, pH_2O, and pCO_2.

B. Blood gas analyses include testing for pH, pO_2, and pCO_2. These tests provide useful information about the respiratory status and the acid-base balance in patients with pulmonary disease or other disorders. (pp. 366, 402)

C. Blood gas analyses do not include testing for pH_2O, pO_2, and pCO_2.

D. Blood gas analyses do not include testing for pH_2O, pO_2, and pH.

26.

A. The alkaline phosphatase level is an enzyme used to evaluate bone activity, not coagulation problems. A prolonged bleeding time may indicate the need for further coagulation testing, such as a platelet count.

B. The acid phosphatase level is an enzyme assay used to evaluate prostate activity, not coagulation problems. A prolonged bleeding time may indicate the need for further coagulation testing, such as a platelet count.

C. A prolonged bleeding time may indicate the need for further coagulation testing, such as a platelet count. (p. 369)

D. Blood urea nitrogen (BUN) test results provide information on kidney function, not coagulation problems as in the bleeding time assay.

27.

A, B, C. One 10-mL syringe with needleless cannula filled with injectable heparinized saline and one 10-mL disposable syringe with needleless cannula are needed for collecting blood through a CVC.

D. One 10-mL syringe with needleless cannula filled with injectable heparinized saline and one 10-mL disposable syringe with needleless cannula are needed for collecting blood through a CVC. (pp. 384–385)

28.

A. The glucose tolerance test (GTT) is a screening test to detect glucose metabolic abnormalities such as diabetes. It is not normally a preoperative screening test.

B. The bleeding-time test is a useful tool for testing platelet plug formation in the capillaries and is used frequently as a preoperative screening test. (p. 368)

C. Blood culture collections are often collected from patients who have fevers of unknown origin. They are used to detect bacterial infections.

D. The lactose tolerance test is run on patients who are experiencing difficulty in digesting milk and other milk products.

29.

A, C, D. The patient needs to follow these guidelines to prepare for the GTT: (1) the patient's carbohydrate intake must be at least 150 grams per day for 3 days before the GTT, (2) the patient should not eat anything for 12 hours before the GTT but should not fast for more than 14 hours before the test, (3) the patient should avoid all possible medications, including corticosteroids, because they will interfere in the GTT, and (4) the patient should avoid exercise for 12 hours before the GTT.

B. The patient needs to follow these guidelines to prepare for the GTT: (1) the patient's carbohydrate intake must be at least 150 grams per day for 3 days before the GTT, (2) the patient should not eat anything for 12 hours before the GTT but should not fast for more than 14 hours before the test, (3) the patient should avoid all possible medications, including corticosteroids, because they will interfere in the GTT, and (4) the patient should avoid exercise for 12 hours before the GTT. (p. 378)

30.

A. The time of collection is much more critical for drugs with shorter half-lives (e.g., gentamicin, tobramycin, and procainamide) than for those with longer half-lives (i.e., phenobarbital, digoxin, and digitoxin). (p. 383)

B, C, D. The time of collection is much more critical for drugs with shorter half-lives (e.g., gentamicin, tobramycin, and procainamide) than for those with longer half-lives (i.e., phenobarbital, digoxin, and digitoxin).

31.

A, B, D. Normally, after an adult patient ingests the 75 or 100 g of glucose in the glucose tolerance test (GTT), the glucose level should return to normal within 2 hours.

C. Normally, after an adult patient ingests the 75 or 100 g of glucose in the glucose tolerance test (GTT), the glucose level should return to normal within 2 hours. (pp. 377, 380)

32.

A. The blood bank phlebotomist does not check the blood donor's glucose value before the blood donation.

B. The blood bank phlebotomist must check the blood donor's hematocrit or hemoglobin value before the blood donation, and it must be no less than 12.5g/dL. (p. 389)

C. The blood bank phlebotomist does not check the blood donor's urine glucose value before the blood donation.

D. The blood bank phlebotomist does not check the blood donor's WBC count value before the blood donation.

33.

A, B, D. The autologous transfusion prevents transfusion-transmitted infectious diseases (e.g., hepatitis C) and eliminates the formation of antibodies in the transfused patient.

C. The autologous transfusion prevents transfusion-transmitted infectious diseases (e.g., hepatitis C) and eliminates the formation of antibodies in the transfused patient. (p. 391)

34.

A. A fasting blood collection is performed in the GTT, and then a standard amount of glucose drink is given to the patient.

B. During the glucose tolerance test (GTT), the patient is required to have numerous urine collections to test for glucose. Therefore, it is imperative for the patient to drink water during the GTT. However, other liquids have to be avoided, since they will interfere in the test results. (p. 377)

C. Sugarless gum must be avoided in the GTT procedure, since it can stimulate digestion and interfere in the test results.

D. All the patient's specimens in the GTT are timed from the minute the patient finishes drinking the glucose solution.

35.

A, B, D. Some otherwise healthy individuals experience difficulty in digesting lactose, a milk sugar. They appear to lack a mucosal lactase enzyme that breaks down the lactose into the simple sugars glucose and galactose.

C. Some otherwise healthy individuals experience difficulty in digesting lactose, a milk sugar. They appear to lack a mucosal lactase enzyme that breaks down the lactose into the simple sugars glucose and galactose. (p. 381)

36.

A, B, C. Iodine may interfere in the blood culture results and therefore must be wiped from the tops of the collection bottles with alcohol.

D. Iodine may interfere in the blood culture results and therefore must be wiped from the tops of the collection bottles with alcohol. (p. 374)

37.

A. A blood pressure cuff (sphygmomanometer) is needed for the Surgicutt procedure.

B. A butterfly-type bandage is needed for the Surgicutt procedure.

C. Disposable gloves are needed for the Surgicutt procedure.

D. A blood pressure cuff (sphygmomanometer), a butterfly-type bandage, and disposable gloves are needed for the Surgicutt procedure. It is a bleeding time procedure, and therefore vacuum blood collection tubes are not required. (p. 370)

38.

A. For therapeutic drug-monitoring collections, a regular cleansing procedure of the venipuncture site is needed.

B. Blood collected for toxicology studies requires a regular cleansing procedure. However, isopropyl alcohol cannot be used as the cleansing solution if blood alcohol levels are being requested.

C. For blood donations, if the donor is not allergic to iodine, a 0.75% PVP-iodine scrub solution is used to scrub the intended phlebotomy site in concentric circles in a 3-inch-diameter area around the venipuncture site. A green soap scrub is used for donors who are allergic to iodine. (p. 486)

D. The lactose tolerance test requires only the usual cleansing procedure for venipuncture collections.

39.

A. CVC is the acronym for central venous catheter, which is also called an intravenous (IV) line.

B. A cannula is a tubular instrument that is used in kidney patients to gain access to venous blood for dialysis or blood collection. (p. 385)

C. A fistula is an artificial shunt in which the vein and artery have been fused through surgery.

D. A cannula is a tubular instrument that is used in kidney patients to gain access to venous blood for dialysis or blood collection.

40.

A, C, D. Therapeutic phlebotomy is the intentional removal of blood in conditions in which

FIGURE 13.1. Arm preparation for collection of blood culture specimens.

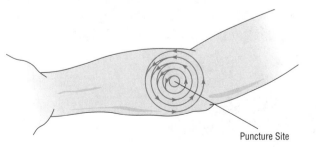

Puncture Site

there is an excessive production of blood cells, as in polycythemia.

B. Therapeutic phlebotomy is the intentional removal of blood in conditions in which there is an excessive production of blood cells, as in polycythemia. (p. 390)

41.

A, B, C. To help minimize the incidence of dizziness, fainting, or other reactions to blood loss, blood donors are encouraged to eat within 4 to 6 hours of donating blood.

D. To help minimize the incidence of dizziness, fainting, or other reactions to blood loss, blood donors are encouraged to eat within 4 to 6 hours of donating blood. (p. 389)

42.

A. Several items must be kept on file on every donor indefinitely, including age.

B. Several items must be kept on file on every donor indefinitely, including a written consent form signed by the donor.

C. Several items must be kept on file on every donor indefinitely, including a record of reason for deferrals.

D. Several items must be kept on file on every donor indefinitely, including age, name, date of birth, a written consent form signed by the donor, and a record of reason for deferrals. The donor, not the donor's parents, consents to his or her own blood collection. (pp. 388–389)

43.

A, C, D. The donor's oral temperature must not exceed 37.5°C (99.5°F).

B. The donor's oral temperature must not exceed 37.5°C (99.5°F). (p. 389)

44.

A, B, D. For the brief physical examination required to determine whether a blood donor is in good health, the donor's systolic blood pressure should measure no higher than 180 mm Hg. People with systolic blood pressures out of this range should be deferred as donors.

C. For the brief physical examination required to determine whether a blood donor is in good health, the donor's systolic blood pressure should measure no higher than 180 mm Hg. People with systolic blood pressures out of this range should be deferred as donors. (p. 389)

45.

A. A false-negative blood culture is more likely to occur if iodine is not wiped from the tops of the blood culture tubes, since iodine may be transferred into the blood culture tube with the needle insertion, causing inhibition of bacterial growth. (p. 374)

B. Usually, indwelling catheters are *not* used for blood culture collections, owing to the possibility of false-positive results that occur from bacterial growth occurring around the catheter.

C. Too much blood collected into the blood culture tube will more likely lead to a false-positive result.

D. If the health care worker palpates the venipuncture site after the site has been prepared without first cleaning the gloved finger, he or she can cause bacterial contamination to the blood collection site, which may lead to a false-positive result.

46.

A. The Allen test is used to compress the patient's ulnar and radial arteries to make certain that these arteries are providing collateral circulation.

B. Blood gas analysis measures pH, pO_2, and pCO_2 but not glucose.

C. To determine whether a patient suffers from lactose intolerance, a physician may order a lactose tolerance test, which involves measuring glucose levels over a 3-hour period. (p. 381)

D. Therapeutic phlebotomy is the intentional removal of blood for therapeutic reasons.

47.

A. The potential blood donor will not be deferred if he or she only weighs 110 pounds.

B. A donor's oral temperature must not exceed 37.5°C. Therefore, this donor's temperature was fine at 37°C.

C. The hematocrit value must be no less than 38% for blood donors. (p. 389)

D. The blood donor's pulse rate should be between 50 and 100 beats per minute.

48.

A. The presence of mild skin disorders, such as a poison ivy rash, does not prohibit an individual from donating unless the lesions are in the antecubital area.

B. Donors with purulent skin lesions, wounds, or severe skin infections should be deferred. The presence of mild skin disorders, such as psoriasis, acne, or a poison ivy rash, does not prohibit an individual from donating unless the lesions are in the antecubital area. (p. 389)

C. The presence of mild skin disorders, such as psoriasis, does not prohibit an individual from donating unless the lesions are in the antecubital area.

D. The presence of mild skin disorders, such as acne, does not prohibit an individual from donating unless the lesions are in the antecubital area.

49.

A, B, D. If the blood donor is allergic to iodine, use soap/acetone alcohol to clean the arm.

C. If the blood donor is allergic to iodine, use soap/acetone alcohol to clean the arm. (pp. 486–487)

50.

A, C, D. A fistula is an artificial shunt in which the vein and artery have been fused through surgery and is a permanent connection tube located in the arm of patients undergoing kidney dialysis.

B. A fistula is an artificial shunt in which the vein and artery have been fused through surgery and is a permanent connection tube located in the arm of patients undergoing kidney dialysis. (p. 385)

14

Elderly, Home, and Long-Term Care Collections

chapter objectives

Upon completion of Chapter 14, the learner is responsible for the following:

➤ List two terms that are synonymous with "point-of-care testing."

➤ Define five physical and/or emotional changes that are associated with the aging process.

➤ Describe how a health care worker should react to physical and emotional changes associated with the elderly.

➤ Identify four analytes whose levels can be determined through point-of-care testing.

➤ Describe the most widely used application of point-of-care testing.

➤ Given the abnormal and normal control values for glucose from a daily run, plot the control values on the appropriate quality control charts.

DIRECTIONS
Each of the questions or incomplete statements below is followed by four suggested answers or completions. Select one answer that is best in each case.

1. Which of the following terms is/are synonymous with "POC testing"?
   A. alternate-site testing
   B. near-patient testing
   C. patient-focused testing
   D. all of the above

2. In point-of-care testing, which of the following conditions can cause erroneous results in glucose testing?
   A. patient having to wait excessively before specimen collection
   B. outdated reagents
   C. calibrators are not used
   D. all of the above

3. The increasing elderly population indicates that point-of-service testing will increase in:
   A. day care centers
   B. homes and rehabilitation centers
   C. commercial pharmacies and health food stores
   D. Internet health sites

4. Hearing loss is common among the elderly and may cause embarrassment or frustration. Which of the following accommodations would be most appropriate and can easily be made to facilitate the specimen collection process?
   A. speak very loudly and forcefully
   B. adjust one's position to speak into the "good" ear

   C. give the patient printed instructions so that verbal communication is not necessary
   D. use a microphone

5. Physical frailties that may affect elderly individuals include:
   A. loss of taste, smell, and feeling
   B. memory loss about taking medications
   C. susceptibility to hypothermia
   D. all of the above

6. Which of the following abbreviations refer(s) to the term "hematocrit"?
   A. Hct, crit
   B. CBC
   C. hemo scan
   D. none of the above

7. Which of the following blood assays can assist in the diagnosis and evaluation of anemia?
   A. Na^+, K^+
   B. hemoglobin and hematocrit
   C. glucose and insulin
   D. all of the above

8. In terms of quality control procedures, "SD" stands for:
   A. short distance
   B. standand deviation
   C. shared diameter
   D. standard dimension

For Questions 9–12, please refer to Figure 14.1, if necessary.

FIGURE 14.1.

Glucose Monitor

QUALITY CONTROL RECORD

PRACTICE NAME

Med Mobile Clinic

INSTRUMENT *Glucose Monitor – Mobile Clinic*

CONTROL LOT# *54539*   EXPIRATION DATE *03/05/05*

DIRECTOR SIGNATURE/DATE:

NAME/LEVEL

Accu Glucose/Normal

TEST	*Glucose *Glucose Monitor*				UNITS	*mg/dl*		
LOWER LIMIT *91*			MEAN *100*		UPPER LIMIT *109*			
DATE	NO.	VALUE	TECH	COMMENT	DATE	NO.	VALUE	TECH	COMMENT

DATE	NO.	VALUE	TECH	COMMENT	DATE	NO.	VALUE	TECH	COMMENT
2/8/04	1	*99*	*KBM*			17			
2/9/04	2	*103*	*KBM*	*prev. maintenance*		18			
2/10/04	3	*100*	*KBM*			19			
2/11/04	4	*100*	*KBM*			20			
2/12/04	5	*105*	*KBM*			21			
2/15/04	6	*97*	*KBM*			22			
2/16/04	7	*95*	*KBM*			23			
2/17/04	8	*96*	*KBM*	*new battery*		24			
2/18/04	9	*103*	*KBM*			25			
2/19/04	10	*100*	*KBM*			26			
2/20/04	11	*103*	*KBM*			27			
2/21/04	12	*97*	*KBM*			28			
	13					29			
	14					30			
	15					31			
	16								

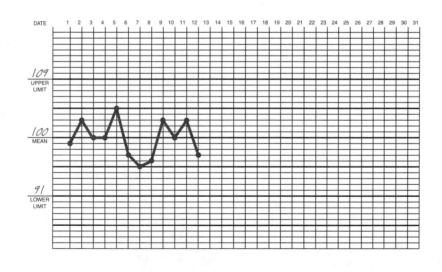

9. Interpretation of a quality control chart is based on the fact that for a normal distribution:
   A. 99% of the values are within 3 SD of the mean
   B. 99% of the values are within 2 SD of the mean
   C. 95% of the values are within 3 SD of the mean
   D. 95% of the values are within 1 SD of the mean

10. Using Figure 14.1, which of the following statements is true?
    A. On day 7, the glucose control was out of the 2 SD control range.
    B. On day 8, the glucose control was the same as the patient's value.
    C. On day 3, the glucose control had a mean value of 100 mg/dL.
    D. On day 1, the glucose control was too low.

11. Using Figure 14.1, identify the tolerance limits for the glucose control.
    A. 91 to 100 mg/dL
    B. 100 to 109 mg/dL
    C. 91 to 109 mg/dL
    D. 96 to 105 mg/dL

12. When referring to a quality control chart like Figure 14.1, what do the comments indicate?
    A. There was a problem on day 2 and day 5.
    B. There was a dead battery on day 5.
    C. Preventative maintenance was properly documented.
    D. all of the above

13. Which of the following is released from the pancreas and has a major effect on blood glucose levels?

A. ACTH
B. insulin
C. thyroxine
D. renin

14. Most rapid methods for glucose testing require:
    A. serum
    B. plasma
    C. skin puncture blood
    D. red blood cells

15. Na^+, K^+, Cl^-, and HCO^- are usually referred to as:
    A. electrolytes
    B. blood gases
    C. hormones
    D. coagulation factors

16. What is troponin 1 and troponin T?
    A. coagulation factors
    B. instruments that are used to test T_4
    C. proteins that are released after a myocardial infarction
    D. electrolytes

17. What should a health care worker do before using reagent strips and/or controls in point-of-care testing?
    A. Check the date that the bottle was opened.
    B. Check the expiration date.
    C. Ensure proper storage temperature.
    D. all of the above

18. Specimen collection in a patient's home may involve unusual positioning of the patient. What is the preferred position or location

from which to collect a blood specimen from a homebound patient?

A. in the bathroom

B. in a comfortable, reclining position

C. seated next to the kitchen table

D. all of the above

19. Transportation requirements for specimens collected from homebound patients include:

A. leakproof containers

B. cooling or heating accommodations

C. timing efficiency in returning to the laboratory

D. all of the above

20. Extra supplies and equipment are needed by home health care workers who collect specimens from homebound patients that are *not* necessary for workers in a hospital. These include:

A. map and wireless phone

B. biohazard container

C. hand disinfectant

D. all of the above

21. Which of the following is an acceptable alternative to hand-washing?

A. cream or foam disinfectants

B. wearing gloves

C. diluted chlorox spray

D. none of the above

22. Which of the following is a debilitating disease causing tremors, particularly in elderly individuals?

A. anemia

B. Parkinson's disease

C. Alzheimer's disease

D. all of the above

23. Emotional factors that are associated with the aging process include:

A. loss of career or retirement

B. loss of spouse

C. depression

D. all of the above

24. Results from point-of-care testing should contain:

A. the exact same information as results from a clinical laboratory

B. the same information as results from a clinical laboratory and a note that the results are from a bedside (or home) rather than the clinical lab

C. a signature from the patient

D. informed consent from the patient

25. Most instruments manufactured for glucose testing have which of the following features?

A. reagent strip or pad

B. reader to record a color reaction

C. buzzer or alarm to alert the health care worker

D. all of the above

26. As compared to a young adult population, when collecting blood from elderly patients, it is important to remember:

A. skin tissue becomes thicker and the phlebotomist must slap the venipuncture area to locate a vein

B. that the angle of penetration of a venipuncture needle needs to be more shallow

C. not to use heat compresses since the skin is thicker than in younger patients

D. that the angle of penetration of a venipuncture needle needs to be deeper since the muscles are thicker

27. Which of the following is NOT a POC blood glucose monitor?
   A. NOVA Biomedical Stat Profile pHOx Plus
   B. INRatio Meter
   C. One Touch Ultra
   D. FreeStyle

28. Which of the following are blood electrolytes that are usually measured by POC?
   A. pH, pO2, and pCO2
   B. sodium, potassium, chloride
   C. PT, INR
   D. troponin T and troponin 1

29. Figure 14.2 shows an instrument for:
   A. urinalysis testing
   B. hematology parameters
   C. chemistry parameters
   D. blood gas measurement

30. Figure 14.3 is a POC analyzer for measurement of:
   A. urinalysis
   B. hemoglobin
   C. blood coagulation
   D. glucose

31. The pancreas produces:
   A. insulin
   B. glucose
   C. cholesterol
   D. hemoglobin

32. Which point-of-care instrument is used to analyze whether a patient has a heart or lung disorder?
   A. HemoCue beta-glucose analyzer
   B. NOVA Biomedical Stat Profile pHOx analyzer
   C. CoaguChek System
   D. HemoCue beta-hemoglobin analyzer

FIGURE 14.2.

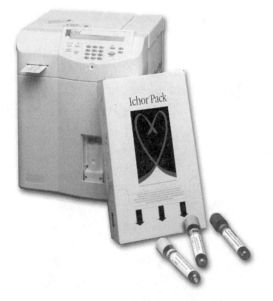

Courtesy of Helena Laboratories, Beaumont, TX

FIGURE 14.3.

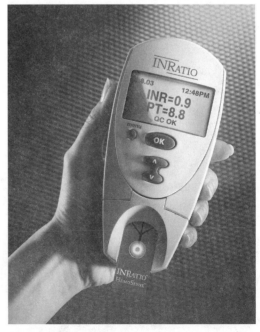

Courtesy of HemoSense, Milpitas, CA

33. In point-of-care testing, the purpose of EQC is to:

    A. calibrate the blood glucose standards

    B. test the instrument's internal and analyte circuits

    C. monitor if the blood sample has been hemolyzed

    D. determine if the blood specimen should be analyzed in the clinical laboratory

34. Which of the following POC instruments uses a microcuvette to measure the analyte?

    A. Accu-Chek

    B. FreeStyle

    C. HemoCue

    D. Nova Biomedical Stat Profile pHOx

35. Which of the following blood analytes is NOT measured through point-of-care testing?

    A. cholesterol

    B. glucose

    C. troponin T or troponin 1

    D. zinc

36. What point-of-care testing procedure is used to test for maintenance of blood glucose levels?

    A. troponin T or troponin 1

    B. prothrombin time

    C. hemoglobin A1c

    D. hemoglobin

37. What should the blood collector do prior to collecting a blood specimen for point-of-care testing?

    A. Make certain that the reagents have been stored at the proper temperature.

    B. Determine if the instrument's battery is working properly.

    C. Check the EQC.

    D. All of the above are correct.

38. The instrument in Figure 14.4 measures:

    A. PCV

    B. PT

    C. RBCs

    D. pCO2

FIGURE 14.4.

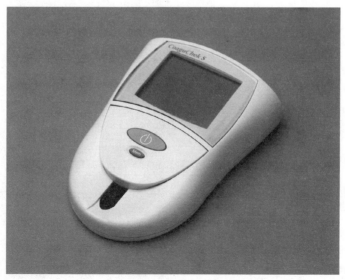

Courtesy of Roche Diagnostics Corp., Indianapolis, IN.

39. The Cardia Status is a POC instrument that measures:
    A. troponin 1, myoglobin, and CK-MB
    B. troponin 1, PT, and myoglobin
    C. myoglobin, INR, and PO2
    D. hemoglobin, troponin 1, and CK-MB

40. The HemoCue beta-glucose analyzer can obtain test results from:
    A. capillary blood
    B. venous blood
    C. arterial blood
    D. all of the above

41. In the development of a quality control record, tolerance limits are determined by pooling the data of laboratory results obtained during what test period?
    A. 5-day test period
    B. 10-day test period
    C. 15-day test period
    D. 30-day test period

42. Which of the following laboratory tests determines whether the blood is too acidic or too alkaline?
    A. Ca^{++}
    B. pH
    C. TCO_2
    D. PCV

43. A less than normal number of erythrocytes is referred to as:
    A. hemoglobin
    B. anemia
    C. diabetes
    D. arthritis

44. POC laboratory testing is the same as:
    A. patient-focused testing

B. bedside testing
C. near-patient testing
D. all of the above

45. For the HemoCue beta-glucose testing procedure,
    A. the dorsal vein is the best location for the blood collection
    B. the first three drops of blood should be wiped away after the incision.
    C. apply a latex-free tourniquet for the procedure
    D. use a safety syringe so that the elderly person's arm will not be damaged from vacuum tubes

46. What blood collection equipment is NOT required for the testing apparatus shown in Figure 14.5?
    A. gauge sponges
    B. tourniquet
    C. gloves
    D. 70% isopropyl alcohol swabs

47. What POC test has been determined to be more accurate than the hematocrit test in diagnosis and treatment of anemia?
    A. RBC count

FIGURE 14.5.

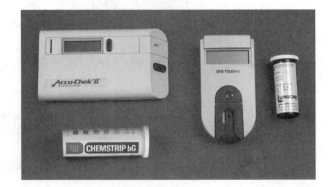

B. WBC count

C. hemoglobin

D. PCV

48. What point-of-care testing procedure is used for a rapid HIV result?

A. Bayer Diagnostics DCA 2000+

B. OraQuick assay

C. HemoCue

D. INRatio Meter

49. For the health care worker who is to perform a glucose POC test, which of the following is *essential* information?

A. what type of blood—from a fingerstick and/or blood from a venipuncture can be used for the POC test

B. the blood type of the patient

C. the patient age group that the blood instrument can be used for

D. both A and C are correct

50. "Quality" in point-of-care testing requires that glucose control material be based on the use of:

A. sterile liquid controls

B. whole blood controls

C. sterile saline controls

D. plasma from pooled patients' blood

51. The POC instruments shown in Figure 14.6 require what body fluid for measurement?

A. whole blood

B. plasma

C. serum

D. all of the above

FIGURE 14.6.

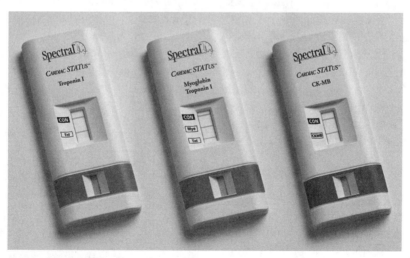

Courtesy of Spectral Diagnostics, Inc., Toronto, Ontario, Canada

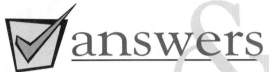

answers & rationales

1.

A, B, C. The demand for point-of-care (POC) testing is increasing because rapid turnaround of laboratory results is necessary for prompt medical decision making. This type of testing occurs at or near the point of direct contact with the patient. Therefore, the terms used for these direct laboratory services include decentralized lab testing, on-site testing, alternate-site testing, near-patient testing, patient-focused testing, and bedside testing.

D. The demand for point-of-care (POC) testing is increasing because rapid turnaround of laboratory results is necessary for prompt medical decision making. This type of testing occurs at or near the point of direct contact with the patient. Therefore, the terms used for these direct laboratory services include decentralized lab testing, on-site testing, alternate-site testing, near-patient testing, patient-focused testing, and bedside testing. (p. 396)

2.

A, B, C. There are many conditions to be careful about and avoid when performing point-of-care glucose testing. These include improper storage of the specimen, contamination of the blood with alcohol, collection of the specimen at the wrong time or after excessive waiting, techniques that are not performed to the manufacturer's recommendations, unclean instruments, outdated or improperly stored reagents, improperly used calibrators and/or controls, and identification or labeling errors.

D. There are many conditions to be careful about and avoid when performing point-of-care glucose testing. These include improper storage of the specimen, contamination of the blood with alcohol, collection of the specimen at the wrong time or after excessive waiting, techniques that are not performed to the manufacturer's recommendations, unclean instruments, outdated or improperly stored reagents, improperly used calibrators and/or controls, and identification or labeling errors. (pp. 399–400, 404)

3.

A. Day care centers are less likely to provide health services involving laboratory testing.

B. Trends in the elderly population indicate that point-of-service testing will increase in patients' homes (home health care), nursing homes (skilled nursing facilities), rehabilitation centers, and other types of long-term care facilities. (p. 397)

C. Commercial pharmacies and health food stores are less likely to offer health services involving laboratory testing.

D. Internet health sites cannot realistically conduct point-of-care testing; however, there are sites that offer advice and/or products that can be used for point-of-care testing.

4.

A. Speaking very loudly and forcefully is not necessary and can be perceived as disrespectful and rude behavior.

B. Hearing loss is common among the elderly. However, not all elderly people are affected by it, and the severity of the problem varies widely. Elderly individuals should be treated with the utmost respect and dignity. Simply repeating the instructions or adjusting one's position to speak into the "good" ear may be all that is needed to ensure the patient's understanding. (p. 397)

C. Giving the patient printed instructions may be a good idea, especially if the degree of deafness is significant, but written instructions should not take the place of a professional, informative dialog. Verbal communication is also necessary because it provides reassurance to the patient and enables the health care worker to check for understanding.

D. Use of a microphone would likely be distracting, embarrassing, and humiliating to the patient.

5.

A, B, C. Physical frailties that may affect elderly individuals include loss of taste, smell, and feeling; memory loss about taking medications; susceptibility to hypothermia; and muscular degeneration.

D. Physical frailties that may affect elderly individuals include loss of taste, smell, and feeling; memory loss about taking medications; susceptibility to hypothermia; and muscular degeneration. (p. 397)

6.

A. The abbreviations "Hct" and "crit" are synonymous with the term "hematocrit." (p. 407)

B. "CBC" is the abbreviation for "complete blood count."

C. "Hemo scan" is not a term that is used for a hematocrit test.

D. "None of the above" is incorrect.

7.

A. Sodium and potassium determinations (Na^+, K^+) are important laboratory tests to evaluate electrolyte balance.

B. Laboratory evaluations of hemoglobin and hematocrit assist in the diagnosis and evaluation of anemia. (p. 407)

C. Glucose and insulin determinations are useful in diagnosing, monitoring, and treating diabetes.

D. "All of the above" is incorrect.

8.

A. "Short distance" is not a quality-control term.

B. "SD" stands for "standard deviation." It is used in quality-control procedures to determine variation from the mean, or the average value that is expected. In a normal distribution of values, 95% of the time the values will be within 2 standard deviations of the mean, and 99% of the values are within 3 standard deviations of the mean. (p. 402)

C. "Shared diameter" is not a quality-control term.

D. "Standard dimension" is not a quality-control term.

For Answers 9–12, please refer to Figure 14.1, if necessary.

9.

A. Interpretation of a quality-control chart is based on the fact that for a normal distribution, 99% of the values are within 3 SD of the mean. (p. 402)

B. In a normal distribution, 99% of the values are not within 2 SD of the mean; only 95% of the values are within 2 SD.

C. In a normal distribution, 99%, not 95%, of the values are within 3 SD of the mean.

D. In a normal distribution, 95% of the values are within 2 SD, not 1 SD of the mean.

10.

A. On day 7, the glucose control was *not* out of the 2 SD control range.

B. This quality control chart is not an evaluation of the patient's glucose level. It only reflects measurements of the glucose control.

C. On day 3, the glucose control had a value of 100 mg/dL, which happens to be the mean value. This is normal and expected. (p. 403)

D. On day 1, the glucose control was *not* too low; it was within 1 SD of the mean.

11.

A. The range 91–100 mg/dL reflects only values within 2 standard deviations *below* the mean.

B. The range 100–109 mg/dL reflects only values within 2 standard deviations *above* the mean.

C. The tolerance limits for the glucose control are from 91 mg/dL (lower limit) to 109 mg/dL (upper limit). (p. 403)

D. This range (96–105 mg/dL) is *within* the tolerance limits of the quality control chart.

12.

A. There was not a problem on day 2 or day 5.

B. There probably was not a dead battery on day 5; rather, there should have been a replaced battery as scheduled by required maintenance.

C. The comments indicate that preventative maintenance was properly documented, and a battery was replaced, as is probably indicated in the required maintenance of the instrument. (p. 403)

D. "All of the above" is incorrect.

13.

A. ACTH (adrenocorticotropic hormone) determinations are useful in assessing endocrine system abnormalities. It is not released from the pancreas.

B. Insulin is released from the pancreas and has a major effect on blood glucose levels. Normally, insulin is released into the bloodstream after meals when glucose levels increase; it causes glucose to be absorbed from the blood into the body tissues where it is used for energy. In patients with diabetes mellitus, glucose is not properly absorbed by the tissues, and the glucose levels within the blood increase. If a patient has an elevated level, he or she can enter a state of metabolic acidosis, which in turn may result in shock and death. (p. 400)

C. Thyroxine (T_4) determinations are used to assess thyroid function. It is not released from the pancreas.

D. Renin determinations are useful in assessing endocrine system abnormalities. It is not released from the pancreas.

FIGURE 14.1. Quality control record.

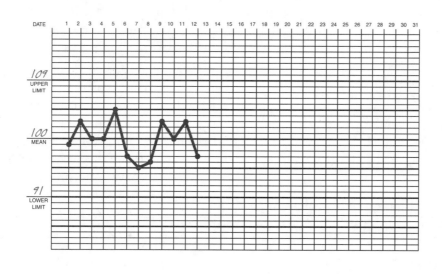

answers & rationales

14.

A. Since serum requires more time to prepare for testing, skin puncture blood is more commonly used for *rapid* procedures.

B. Plasma may also be used; however, skin puncture blood provides a more immediate sample for testing.

C. Most rapid methods for glucose testing require skin puncture blood. (p. 400)

D. Red blood cells alone are not used for rapid glucose testing.

15.

A. Na$^+$, K$^+$, Cl$^-$, and HCO$^-$ are usually referred to as electrolytes. (p. 405)

B. Blood gas analyses include measurement of the partial pressure of oxygen, carbon dioxide, and blood pH.

C. Hormone levels are usually associated with evaluation of the endocrine or reproductive systems.

D. Coagulation factors evaluate bleeding and clotting potential.

16.

A. Troponin T and troponin 1 are not coagulation factors.

B. Troponin T and troponin 1 are not instruments that are used to test T$_4$.

C. Troponin T and troponin 1 are proteins that are released after a myocardial infarction. (p. 405)

D. Troponin T and troponin 1 are not electrolytes.

17.

A, B, C. Point-of-care testing requires careful attention to quality control measures and details. Before using reagent strips and/or controls in point-of-care testing, a health care worker should check the date that the bottle was opened, check the expiration date, and ensure proper storage temperature.

D. Point-of-care testing requires careful attention to quality control measures and details. Before using reagent strips and/or controls in point-of-care testing, a health care worker should check the date that the bottle was opened, check the expiration date, and ensure proper storage temperature. (p. 404)

18.

A. In performing specimen collection procedures in the home, it is important for the health care worker to identify where the bathroom is in relation to the patient. This way, the health care worker can easily wash hands or perhaps even use clean towels if available.

B. The preferred position/location from which to collect a blood specimen from a homebound patient is in a comfortable, reclining position so that the patient does not fall if he or she faints. (p. 398)

C. The preferred position is in a reclining one for safety sake. When a patient is seated next to the kitchen table, there is a greater possibility of injury if he or she falls out of a chair after fainting. Often, there is no one else who can assist the health care worker if this scenario occurs.

D. "All of the above" is incorrect.

19.

A, B, C. Transportation requirements for specimens collected from homebound patients include use of leakproof containers, ensuring appropriate temperature requirements by using cooling or heating instruments, and careful attention to timing when returning specimens to the laboratory for testing. Delays should be well documented.

D. Transportation requirements for specimens collected from homebound patients include use of leakproof containers, ensuring appropriate temperature requirements by using cooling or heating instruments, and careful attention to timing when returning specimens to the laboratory for testing. Delays should be well documented. (p. 398)

20.

A. Extra supplies and equipment needed by home health care workers who collect specimens from homebound patients that are *not* necessary for workers in a hospital are a map and a wireless phone. The map prevents the worker from getting lost in route to or from the home. The phone is helpful under difficult or emergency circumstances. (p. 398)

B. A biohazard container is necessary both for workers in a hospital and in the home.

C. Hand disinfectant or hand-washing is necessary both for workers in a hospital and in the home.

D. "All of the above" is incorrect.

21.

A. Using cream or foam disinfectants is an acceptable alternative to hand-washing. This may be particularly helpful in the home setting if conditions are not very clean. (p. 398)

B. Wearing gloves should always occur and is not a substitute for hand-washing.

C. Using diluted chlorox spray on one's hands is not a good substitute for hand-washing.

D. "None of the above" is incorrect.

22.

A. Anemia is not necessarily associated with the aging process and does not cause tremors.

B. Parkinson's disease is a debilitating disease causing tremors, particularly in elderly individuals. (p. 397)

C. Alzheimer's disease is also associated with the aging process; however, it affects the mind.

D. "All of the above" is incorrect.

23.

A, B, C. Emotional factors that are associated with the aging process include loss of career or retirement, loss of spouse or close friends, and depression or anger at life.

D. Emotional factors that are associated with the aging process include loss of career or retirement, loss of spouse or close friends, and depression or anger at life. (p. 397)

24.

A. Results should contain the exact same information as results from a clinical laboratory in addition to a note about the site of testing (bedside or home testing).

B. Results from point-of-care testing should contain the same information as results from a clinical laboratory plus a note that the results are from a bedside (or home) rather than the clinical laboratory. (p. 401)

C. A signature from the patient is not necessary on the test results.

D. Informed consent from the patient is needed but not on the results of the laboratory test.

25.

A, B, C. Most instruments manufactured for POC glucose testing have a reagent strip or pad, a reader to record a color reaction on the strip/pad, and a buzzer or alarm to alert the health care worker that it is time to read the result. Timing of the reaction is critical.

D. Most instruments manufactured for POC glucose testing have a reagent strip or pad, a reader to record a color reaction on the strip/pad, and a buzzer or alarm to alert the health care worker that it is time to read the result. Timing of the reaction is critical. (pp. 400–401)

26.

A. As compared to a young adult population, when collecting blood from elderly patients, it is important to remember that their skin tissue becomes thinner and thus, the arm must not be slapped since it may cause bruising.

B. As compared to a young adult population, when collecting blood from elderly patients, it is important that the angle of penetration of a venipuncture needle may need to be more shallow since the muscles become smaller. (p. 397)

C. As compared to a young adult population, when collecting blood from elderly patients, it is important to warm the venipuncture site since the elderly are more susceptible to cold temperatures.

D. As compared to a young adult population, when collecting blood from elderly patients, it is important that the angle of penetration of a venipuncture needle may need to be more shallow since the muscles become smaller.

27.

A. The NOVA Biomedical Stat Profile pHOx Plus provides analysis for blood gases, electrolytes, and glucose.

B. The INRatio Meter is used for blood co-agulation monitoring, not glucose testing. (pp. 406–408)

C. The One Touch Ultra is a POC blood glucose monitor.

D. The FreeStyle is a POC blood glucose monitor.

28.

A. pH, pO2, and pCO2 are blood gas measurements usually performed by POC.

B. Sodium, potassium, and chloride are blood electrolytes usually measured by POC. (p. 405)

C. PT and INR are blood coagulation measurements.

D. Troponin T and troponin 1 are assays to detect health damage.

29.

A. Figure 14.2 is not an instrument for urinalysis testing.

B. Figure 14.2 shows the Ichor automated cell counter (Helena Laboratories, Beaumont, TX), an instrument for hematology analysis in acute adult and pediatric patient management. (pp. 408, 410)

C. Figure 14.2 is not an instrument for chemistry parameters.

D. Figure 14.2 is not an instrument for blood gas measurement.

FIGURE 14.2. Ichor automated cell counter.

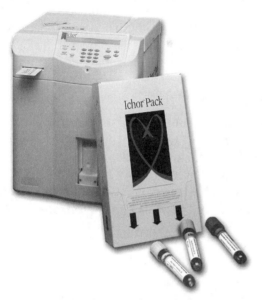

Courtesy of Helena Laboratories, Beaumont, TX

32.

A, C, D. The NOVA Biomedical Stat Profile pHOx analyzer measures blood gases (pH, pCO2, pO2) that can detect whether a patient has a heart or lung disorder.

B. The NOVA Biomedical Stat Profile pHOx analyzer measures blood gases (pH, pCO2, pO2) that can detect whether a patient has a heart or lung disorder. (p. 402)

33.

A, C, D. In point-of-care testing, the purpose of "electronic quality control" (EQC) is to test the instrument's internal and analyte circuits.

B. In point-of-care testing, the purpose of "electronic quality control" (EQC) is to test the instrument's internal and analyte circuits. (p. 401)

30.

A. Figure 14.3 is not a POC analyzer for urinalysis.

B. Figure 14.3 is not a POC analyzer for measurement of hemoglobin.

C. Figure 14.3 is a POC analyzer for measurement of Prothrombin time (PT) and INRatio to detect blood coagulation problems. (pp. 406, 408)

D. Figure 14.3 is a POC analyzer for measurement of Prothrombin time (PT) and INRatio to detect blood coagulation problems.

31.

A. Insulin is a chemical that is released into the bloodstream by the pancreas when glucose levels in the blood increase. (p. 400)

B, C, D. Insulin is a chemical that is released into the bloodstream by the pancreas when glucose levels in the blood increase.

FIGURE 14.3. INRatio meter.

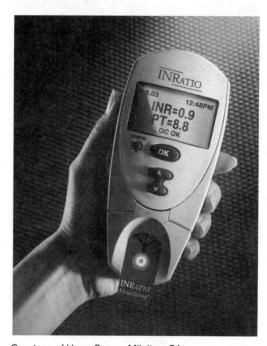

Courtesy of HemoSense, Milpitas, CA

34.

A, B, D. The HemoCue beta-glucose analyzer and HemoCue beta-Hemoglobin System both use a microcuvette to measure the analyte.

C. The HemoCue beta-glucose analyzer and HemoCue beta-Hemoglobin System both use a microcuvette to measure the analyte. (pp. 398–399, 409)

35.

A. Cholesterol can be measured through point-of-care testing.

B. Glucose can be measured through point-of-care testing.

C. Troponin T or troponin 1 can be measured through point-of-care testing.

D. Cholesterol, glucose, troponin 1, and troponin T can all be measured through point-of-care testing. Zinc is a trace element that requires special collection in a trace element (royal blue) vacuum collection tube and special testing procedures. (pp. 398, 405, 408, 480)

36.

A. Troponin T or troponin 1 is used to detect heart damage, not maintenance of blood glucose levels.

B. Prothrombin time is a coagulation test to determine if a patient has a blood clotting disorder.

C. Hemoglobin A1c is a procedure to test for maintenance of blood glucose levels. (p. 409)

D. Hemoglobin testing is used to aid in the diagnosis and evaluation of anemia and other blood abnormalities.

37.

A, B, C. Prior to collecting a blood specimen for point-of-care testing, the blood collector should: (1) make certain that the reagents have been stored at the proper temperature; (2) determine if the instrument's battery is working properly, and (3) check the "electronic quality control" (EQC).

D. Prior to collecting a blood specimen for point-of-care testing, the blood collector should: (1) make certain that the reagents have been stored at the proper temperature; (2) determine if the instrument's battery is working properly, and (3) check the "electronic quality control" (EQC). (pp. 401, 404).

38.

A. Figure 14.4 does not measure PCV.

B. Figure 14.4 is the CoaguChek System that measures prothrombin time (PT). (p. 406)

C. Figure 14.4 does not measure RBCs.

D. Figure 14.4 does not measure pCO_2.

39.

A. The CardiaStatus is a cardiac POC instrument that can be used to measure troponin 1, myoglobin, and CK-MB. (p. 405)

B, C, D. The CardiaStatus is a cardiac POC instrument that can be used to measure troponin 1, myoglobin, and CK-MB.

40.

A, B, C. The HemoCue beta-glucose analyzer can obtain test results from capillary, venous, or arterial whole blood.

D. The HemoCue beta-glucose analyzer can obtain test results from capillary, venous, or arterial whole blood. (p. 401)

FIGURE 14.4. CoaguChek System.

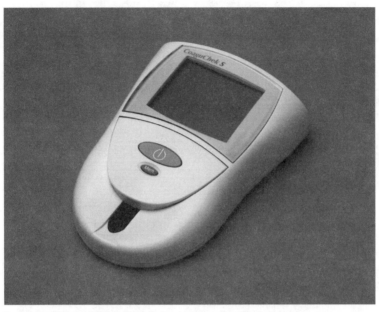

Courtesy of Roche Diagnostics Corp., Indianapolis, IN.

41.

A, B, C. In the development of a quality control record, tolerance limits are determined by pooling the data of laboratory results obtained during a 30-day test period.

D. In the development of a quality control record, tolerance limits are determined by pooling the data of laboratory results obtained during a 30-day test period. (p. 402)

42.

A, C, D. The blood pH determines whether the blood is too acidic or too alkaline.

B. The blood pH determines whether the blood is too acidic or too alkaline. (p. 402)

43.

A. Hemoglobin are the molecules that carry oxygen and carbon dioxide in the RBCs.

B. A less than normal number of erythrocytes is referred to as anemia. (p. 407)

C. Diabetes is a metabolic disease in which glucose is not utilized normally in the body.

D. Arthritis is a joint disorder that affects mainly older people.

44.

A, B, C. Point-of-care (POC) testing is the same as patient-focused testing, bedside testing, alternate site testing, and near-patient testing.

D. Point-of-care (POC) testing is the same as patient-focused testing, bedside testing, alternate site testing, and near-patient testing. (p. 396)

45.

A, C, D. The HemoCue beta-glucose testing procedure requires that the first three drops of blood be wiped away after a skin puncture.

B. The HemoCue beta-glucose testing procedure requires that the first three drops of blood be wiped away after a skin puncture. (pp. 398–399)

46.

A. The glucose meters and blood chemistry strips shown in Figure 14.5 use blood from skin puncture techniques or a flushed heparin line. Thus, gauge sponges are needed.

B. The glucose meters and blood chemistry strips shown in Figure 14.5 use blood from skin puncture techniques or a flushed heparin line. Thus, gauge sponges, gloves, and 70% isopropyl alcohol swabs are needed, but a tourniquet is not needed for skin puncture or IV line collection. (pp. 400–401)

C. The glucose meters and blood chemistry strips shown in Figure 14.5 use blood from skin puncture techniques or a flushed heparin line. Thus, gloves are needed.

D. The glucose meters and blood chemistry strips shown in Figure 14.5 use blood from skin puncture techniques or a flushed heparin line. Thus, 70% isopropyl alcohol swabs are needed.

FIGURE 14.5. Use of glucose meters.

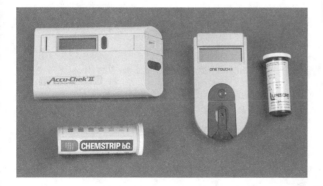

47.

A, B, D. The hemoglobin test has been determined by the American Medical Association (AMA) to be more accurate than the hematocrit test in diagnosis and treatment of anemia.

C. The hemoglobin test has been determined by the American Medical Association (AMA) to be more accurate than the hematocrit test in diagnosis and treatment of anemia. (p. 407)

48.

A, C, D. The rapid HIV point-of-care test is the OraQuick assay.

B. The rapid HIV point-of-care test is the OraQuick assay. (p. 409)

49.

A, B, C. For the health care worker who is to perform a glucose POC test, he or she needs to know what type of blood—blood from a finger stick and/or blood from venipuncture—can be used to perform glucose determination with the POC instrument and the patient age group that the blood instrument can be used for.

D. For the health care worker who is to perform a glucose POC test, he or she needs to know what type of blood—blood from a finger stick and/or blood from venipuncture—can be used to perform glucose determination with the POC instrument and the patient age group that the blood instrument can be used for. (pp. 400–401)

50.

A, C, D. "Quality" in point-of-care testing requires that glucose control material be based on the use of whole blood controls similar to the patient's specimen in order to determine if the analytic system is working properly.

B. "Quality" in point-of-care testing requires that glucose control material be based on the use of whole blood controls similar to the patient's specimen in order to determine if the analytic system is working properly. (p. 401)

51.

A, B, C. The POC instruments shown in Figure 14.6 are used for cardiac point-of-care testing and can use whole blood, plasma, or serum from a patient to be tested.

D. The POC instruments shown in Figure 14.6 are used for cardiac point-of-care testing and can use whole blood, plasma, or serum from a patient to be tested. (p. 405)

FIGURE 14.6. Spectral CardiaSTATus.

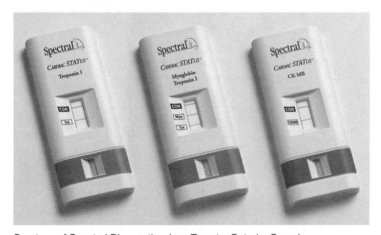

Courtesy of Spectral Diagnostics, Inc., Toronto, Ontario, Canada

CHAPTER

15

Urinalysis, Body Fluid, and Other Specimens

chapter objectives

Upon completion of Chapter 15, the learner is responsible for the following:

➤ Identify the types of body fluid specimens, other than blood, that are analyzed in the clinical laboratory and the correct procedures for collecting and/or transporting these specimens to the laboratory.

➤ Identify the various types of specimens collected for micro-biological, throat, and nasopharyngeal cultures and the protocol that health care workers must follow when transporting these specimens.

➤ List the types of patient specimens that are needed for gastric and sweat chloride analyses.

➤ List three types of urine specimen collections and differentiate the uses of the urine specimens obtained from these collections.

DIRECTIONS
Each of the questions or incomplete statements below is followed by four suggested answers or completions. Select one answer that is best in each case.

1. BUN test measures the amount of what in the blood and can detect problems with the urinary system?
   A. creatinine
   B. HCG
   C. urea
   D. TSH

2. For the urinary pregnancy test, the preferred urine specimen is a:
   A. 2-hour urine collection
   B. 24-hour urine sample
   C. random urine sample
   D. clean-catch midstream sample

3. Which of the following is obtained through a lumbar puncture?
   A. pleural fluid
   B. cerebrospinal fluid
   C. synovial fluid
   D. peritoneal fluid

4. Nasopharyngeal culture collections may be used to diagnose:
   A. whooping cough
   B. *Salmonella* infection
   C. *Shigella* infection
   D. *Crytococcus* infection

5. Fluid composed of products formed in various male reproductive organs is referred to as:
   A. pleural fluid
   B. seminal fluid
   C. synovial fluid
   D. cerebrospinal fluid

6. The ColoScreen-ES test is run on
   A. synovial fluid
   B. feces
   C. urine
   D. CSF

7. Which of the following types of urine specimens is the "cleanest," or least contaminated?
   A. first morning specimen
   B. timed specimen
   C. midstream specimen
   D. random specimen

8. Creatinine clearance is determined through use of:
   A. urine specimens
   B. pericardial fluid specimens
   C. synovial fluid
   D. CSF specimens

9. Amniotic fluid can be found:
   A. around the lungs
   B. surrounding the heart
   C. around the fetus in the uterus
   D. surrounding the liver, the pancreas, and other parts of the gastrointestinal area

10. A urine C & S should be performed on a:
    A. random urine sample
    B. clean-catch midstream sample
    C. routine urine sample
    D. 24-hour urine specimen

11. Peritoneal fluid is located:
    A. around the lungs
    B. in the joints
    C. in the abdomen
    D. in the sac around the heart

12. A 24-hour urine specimen is usually collected to test for:
    A. hormones
    B. glucose
    C. creatine kinase
    D. bacteria

13. Pericardial fluid is collected from the
    A. abdomen
    B. sac around the heart
    C. joints
    D. sac around the lungs

14. Skin tests are used to determine whether a patient has ever had contact with:
    A. a particular antibody and has produced antigens to that antibody
    B. a particular antigen and has produced antibodies to that antigen
    C. the disease leukemia
    D. the disease polycythemia

15. The fluid collected from a joint cavity is:
    A. peritoneal fluid
    B. pleural fluid
    C. abdominal fluid
    D. synovial fluid

16. Throat cultures are most commonly obtained to determine the presence of:
    A. *Neisseria* infection
    B. *Streptococcus* infection
    C. *Staphylococcus* infection
    D. *Bacillus* infection

17. The best site for a sweat chloride test on a child is the:
    A. arm
    B. hand
    C. leg
    D. finger

18. What type of urine specimen is needed to detect an infection?
    A. random
    B. clean-catch
    C. routine
    D. 24-hour

19. Which of the following types of specimens is most frequently collected for analysis?
    A. amniotic fluid
    B. urine
    C. CSF
    D. pericardial fluid

20. The O & P analysis is requested on:
    A. CSF specimens
    B. amniotic fluid specimens
    C. fecal specimens
    D. synovial fluid specimens

21. The occult blood analysis is frequently requested on:
    A. CSF specimens
    B. fecal specimens
    C. throat cultures
    D. seminal fluid specimens

22. Ketosis is frequently associated with:
    A. liver disease
    B. diabetes mellitus
    C. chemical poisoning
    D. infection

23. Which of the following can be used in children and infants to diagnose whooping cough?
    A. Hollander test
    B. nasopharyngeal culture
    C. O & P test
    D. sweat chloride test

24. The sweat chloride test is used to diagnose:
    A. cerebral palsy
    B. multiple sclerosis
    C. cystic fibrosis
    D. diabetes mellitus

25. What is the specimen of choice for drug abuse testing?
    A. CSF
    B. gastric fluid
    C. synovial fluid
    D. urine

26. The Keo-Diastix strip is used to test:
    A. cerebrospinal fluid
    B. urine
    C. amniotic fluid
    D. fecal specimens

27. For the TB skin test, the tuberculin syringe should be held at what angle for administration of the antigen?
    A. 5 degrees
    B. 10 degrees
    C. 20 degrees
    D. 45 degrees

28. Figure 15.1 is illustrating:
    A. the TB skin test
    B. sweat chloride test
    C. allergy skin test
    D. glucose skin puncture test

29. Figure 15.2 is illustrating a collection procedure for:
    A. breath analysis for peptic ulcers
    B. gastric analysis
    C. sweat chloride procedure
    D. *Streptococcus pyogenes*

FIGURE 15.1.

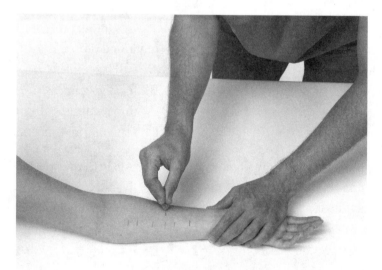

Source: Andy Crawford/Dorling Kindersley Media Library.

FIGURE 15.2.

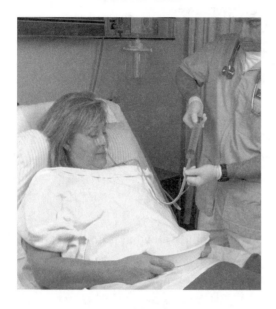

30. Occult quantities of blood refer to:
    A. large quantities of blood
    B. small quantities of blood
    C. invisible quantities of blood
    D. hemolytic quantities of blood

31. The ColoScreen-ES test is used to detect:
    A. occult blood
    B. hemolytic blood
    C. fungal infections
    D. bacterial infections

32. Urine is most concentrated:
    A. in the afternoon
    B. in the evening
    C. after dinner
    D. in the morning

33. Glycosuria is:
    A. presence of glucose in urine
    B. presence of glycogen in urine
    C. presence of glucose in blood
    D. presence of glycogen in cerebrospinal
       fluid.

34. What is the first step performed in the clean-catch midstream urine collection for women?
    A. Hold the skin folds apart with one hand and urinate into the collection container.
    B. After washing her hands, the patient should separate the skin folds around the urinary opening and clean this area.
    C. The woman should urinate into the specially cleaned urine container.
    D. The woman needs to separate the skin folds around the urinary opening and urinate into the specially cleaned urine container.

35. In Figure 15.3, the patient is collecting:
    A. a sputum specimen
    B. a throat culture specimen
    C. a wound specimen
    D. a nasopharyngeal culture specimen

36. Which of the following is used to detect cystic fibrosis?
    A. breath analysis
    B. sweat chloride test
    C. gastric analysis
    D. O & P

FIGURE 15.3.

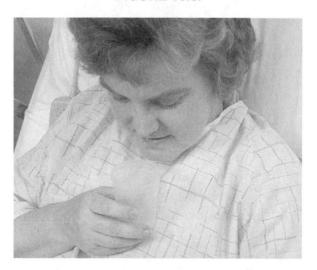

37. The *H.pylori* test is:
    A. gastric analysis
    B. breath analysis
    C. the sweat chloride test
    D. the ColoScreen-ES test

38. What is the name of the disorder that affects the exocrine glands and affects the lungs, upper respiratory tract, liver, and pancreas?
    A. diabetes mellitus
    B. cystic fibrosis
    C. pneumonia
    D. diabetes insipidus

39. When hemoglobin is detected on the urine dipstick from a patient's urine specimen, this indicates:
    A. glycosuria
    B. blood destruction
    C. high chloride levels
    D. leukocytes in the urine

40. Glucose-level determinations for diabetes mellitus testing should occur on what type of urine specimen collection?
    A. random specimen
    B. fasting specimen
    C. clean-catch specimen
    D. first urine of the morning specimen

41. Which of the following are included in the physical analysis of a urine sample?
    A. red blood cells
    B. hemoglobin
    C. transparency
    D. ketones

42. The presence of bilirubin in the urine may be associated with:
    A. diabetes mellitus
    B. malaria
    C. liver disease
    D. infection in the kidney

43. Which of the following is used as an indicator of "clearance" in how the kidney is able to remove and filter analytes from the body?
    A. creatinine
    B. creatine
    C. hemoglobin
    D. glucose

44. Which of the following is collected through a lumbar puncture?
    A. peritoneal fluid
    B. CSF
    C. seminal fluid
    D. pleural fluid

45. The second tube of CSF collected through a spinal tap is used for:
    A. clinical chemistry
    B. serological testing
    C. clinical microbiology testing
    D. microscopic analysis

46. When instructing the patient to collect a 24-hour urine specimen, what time period is recommended for discontinuation of medications preceding the urine collection?
    A. 4 to 12 hours
    B. 12 to 24 hours
    C. 24 to 36 hours
    D. 48 to 72 hours

47. Fecal specimens are sometimes collected in order to detect:
    A. *Haemophilus influenzae*
    B. *Salmonella species*

C. *Corynebacterium diphtheriae*

D. *Mycobacterium tuberculosis*

48. The test used to diagnose whooping cough and pneumonia is:

A. creatinine clearance

B. nasopharyngeal culture

C. O & P

D. breath analysis

49. Fluid from the lungs containing pus is:

A. seminal fluid

B. amniotic fluid

C. sputum

D. synovial fluid

50. In the gastric analysis procedure, what is injected into the patient as a stimulant?

A. creatinine

B. histamine

C. hemoglobin

D. pilocarpine hydrochloric acid

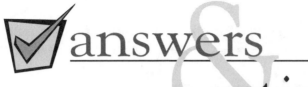
answers & rationales

answers & rationales

1.

A. BUN (Blood Urea Nitrogen) measures urea, not creatinine.

B. BUN (Blood Urea Nitrogen) measures urea, not HCG.

C. BUN (Blood Urea Nitrogen) measures urea in the blood and is a procedure to determine how well the urinary system is functioning. (p. 416)

D. BUN (Blood Urea Nitrogen) measures urea, not TSH.

2.

A, B, D. A random urine sample (UA) is the specimen of choice for a urinary pregnancy test.

C. A random urine sample (UA) is the specimen of choice for a urinary pregnancy test. (pp. 414–417)

3.

A. Pleural fluid is obtained from the lung cavity.

B. Cerebrospinal fluid (CSF) is obtained by a physician through a spinal tap or lumbar puncture. (p. 419)

C. Synovial fluid is obtained aseptically from joint cavities.

D. Peritoneal fluid is obtained from the abdominal cavity.

4.

A. Nasopharyngeal culture collections may be used to diagnose whooping cough. (p. 423)

B. Nasopharyngeal culture collections are not used to diagnose *Salmonella* infection.

C. Nasopharyngeal culture collections are not used to diagnose *Shigella* infection.

D. Nasopharyngeal culture collections are not used to diagnose *Crytococcus* infection.

5.

A. Pleural fluid is in the lungs.

B. Seminal fluid is composed of products formed in various male reproductive organs. (p. 421)

C. Synovial fluid is in the joints.

D. Cerebrospinal fluid is in the spinal column and contains numerous analytes, including protein, glucose, and chloride.

6.

A. The Colo-Screen ES test is not performed on synovial fluid.

B. The Colo-Screen ES test is performed on stool (feces) specimens. (p. 421)

C. The Colo-Screen ES test is not performed on urine.

D. The Colo-Screen ES test is not performed on CSF.

7.

A, B, D. The midstream, or clean-catch, specimen is the "cleanest" or least-contaminated urine specimen.

C. The midstream, or clean-catch, specimen is the "cleanest" or least-contaminated urine specimen. (pp. 416–418)

8.

A. The creatinine clearance used to determine kidney damage is based on results from urine and blood specimens. (p. 416)

B. The creatinine clearance used to determine kidney damage is not based on results from pericardial fluid specimens.

C. The creatinine clearance used to determine kidney damage is not based on results from synovial fluid specimens.

D. The creatinine clearance used to determine kidney damage is not based on results from CSF specimens.

9.

A. Pleural fluid is in the lung cavity.

B. Pericardial fluid surrounds the heart.

C. Amniotic fluid surrounds the fetus in the uterus. (p. 421)

D. Peritoneal fluid is within the abdominal cavity.

10.

A, C, D. A urine culture and sensitivity (C & S) test requires a clean-catch midstream urine collection to avoid contamination.

B. A urine culture and sensitivity (C & S) test requires a clean-catch midstream urine collection to avoid contamination. (p. 416)

11.

A. Pleural fluid is located in the lung cavity.

B. Synovial fluid is found in the joints.

C. Peritoneal fluid is located in the abdomen. (p. 422)

D. Pericardial fluid is located in the sac around the heart.

12.

A. A 24-hour urine specimen is usually collected to test for hormone studies or the creatinine clearance. (p. 416)

B, C, D. A 24-hour urine specimen is usually collected to test for hormone studies or the creatinine clearance.

13.

A. Peritoneal fluid is collected from the abdominal cavity.

B. Pericardial fluid is collected from the sac around the heart. (p. 422)

C. Synovial fluid is collected from the abdominal cavity.

D. Pleural fluid is collected from the sac around the lungs.

14.

A, C, D. Skin tests are used to determine whether a patient has ever had contact with a particular antigen and has produced antibodies to that antigen.

B. Skin tests are used to determine whether a patient has ever had contact with a particular antigen and has produced antibodies to that antigen. (p. 425)

15.

A. Peritoneal fluid is collected from the abdominal cavity.

B. Pleural fluid is collected from the lung cavity.

C. The fluid collected from a joint cavity is synovial fluid.

D. The fluid collected from a joint cavity is synovial fluid. (p. 422)

16.

A, C, D. Throat cultures are most commonly obtained to determine the presence of a streptococcal infection.

B. Throat cultures are most commonly obtained to determine the presence of a streptococcal infection. (p. 423)

17.

A, B, D. To perform the sweat chloride test on a child, the health care worker should choose a site with a large surface area; the best site is the leg.

C. To perform the sweat chloride test on a child, the health care worker should choose a site with a large surface area; the best site is the leg. (p. 428)

18.

A, C, D. The clean-catch urine specimen is used to detect the presence or absence of infecting organisms. Therefore, the specimen is collected in such a manner as to avoid contamination by bacteria on the external genital areas.

B. The clean-catch urine specimen is used to detect the presence or absence of infecting organisms. Therefore, the specimen is collected in such a manner as to avoid contamination by bacteria on the external genital areas. (p. 416)

19.

A, C, D. Routine urinalysis is one of the most frequently requested laboratory procedures because it can provide a useful indication of body health.

B. Routine urinalysis is one of the most frequently requested laboratory procedures because it can provide a useful indication of body health. (p. 414)

20.

A. CSF specimens are not commonly collected to detect parasites, such as ova and parasites (O & P).

B. Amniotic fluid specimens are not commonly collected to detect parasites, such as ova and parasites (O & P).

C. Stool (fecal) specimens are commonly collected to detect parasites, such as ova and parasites (O & P), enteric disease organisms, and viruses. (p. 421)

D. Synovial fluid specimens are not commonly collected to detect parasites, such as ova and parasites (O & P).

21.

A. Laboratory determination of occult (invisible) blood is not requested on CSF specimens.

B. Laboratory determination of occult (invisible) blood in feces can assist in the confirmation of the presence of blood in black stools and be helpful in detecting gastrointestinal tract lesions and colorectal cancer. (p. 421)

C and D. Laboratory determination of occult (invisible) blood is not requested on throat cultures or seminal fluid specimens.

22.

A, C, D. Ketosis (presence of ketone bodies in urine) is frequently detected in patients who have diabetes mellitus.

B. Ketosis (presence of ketone bodies in urine) is frequently detected in patients who have diabetes mellitus. (p. 415)

23.

A, C, D. A nasopharyngeal culture is often performed to detect carrier states of bacteria such as *Haemophilus influenzae* and *Staphylococcus aureus.* In children and infants, this type of culture can be used to diagnose whooping cough, croup, and pneumonia.

B. A nasopharyngeal culture is often performed to detect carrier states of bacteria such as *Haemophilus influenzae* and *Staphylococcus aureus.* In children and infants, this type of culture can be used to diagnose whooping cough, croup, and pneumonia. (p. 423)

24.

A. The sweat chloride test is not used in the diagnosis of cerebral palsy.

B. The sweat chloride test is not used in the diagnosis of multiple sclerosis.

C. The sweat chloride test is used in the diagnosis of cystic fibrosis. Cystic fibrosis is a disorder of the exocrine glands. (p. 427)

D. The sweat chloride test is not used in the diagnosis of diabetes mellitus.

25.

A. CSF is not the specimen of choice for drug abuse testing.

B. Gastric fliud is not the specimen of choice for drug abuse testing.

C. Synovial fluid is not the specimen of choice for drug abuse testing.

D. Urine is the specimen of choice for drug abuse testing. The end product metabolites of drugs, as well as the drugs, are excreted in the urine. (p. 416)

26.

A. The Keo-Diastrix strip is not used to test CSF.

B. The Keo-Diastrix strip is used to test urine for ketone bodies. (p. 417)

C. The Keo-Diastrix strip is not used to test amniotic fluid.

D. The Keo-Diastrix strip is not used to test fecal specimens.

27.

A, B, D. For the TB skin test, the tuberculin syringe should be held at an angle of 20 degrees for administration of the antigen.

C. For the TB skin test, the tuberculin syringe should be held at an angle of 20 degrees for administration of the antigen. (p. 425)

FIGURE 15.1. Allergy skin testing.

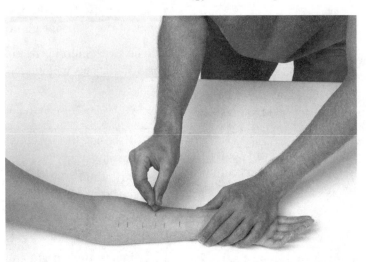

Source: Andy Crawford/Dorling Kindersley Media Library.

28.

A. Figure 15.1 is not illustrating the TB skin test.

B. Figure 15.1 is not illustrating the sweat chloride test.

C. Figure 15.1 is illustrating the allergy skin test that is performed on the patient's forearm or back using a common procedure called the prick technique. (pp. 425–426)

D. Figure 15.1 is not illustrating the glucose skin puncture test.

29.

A, C, D. Figure 15.2 is illustrating a collection procedure for gastric analysis in which the patient is intubated to obtain the gastric contents.

B. Figure 15.2 is illustrating a collection procedure for gastric analysis in which the patient is intubated to obtain the gastric contents. (pp. 426–427)

30.

A. Occult quantities of blood does not refer to large quantities of blood.

B. Occult quantities of blood does not refer to small quantities of blood.

C. Occult quantities of blood refer to invisible quantities of blood that may occur in fecal specimens. (p. 421)

FIGURE 15.2. Aspirating gastric contents from the patient.

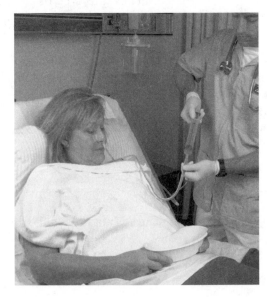

D. Occult quantities of blood does not refer to hemolytic quantities of blood.

31.

A. The ColoScreen-ES test is used to detect occult blood in feces. (p. 421)

B. The ColoScreen-ES test is not used to detect hemolytic blood.

C. The ColoScreen-ES test is not used to detect fungal infections.

D. The ColoScreen-ES test is not used to detect bacterial infections.

32.

A. Urine is most concentrated in the morning.

B. Urine is most concentrated in the morning.

C. Urine is most concentrated in the morning.

D. Urine is most concentrated in the morning. (p. 418)

33.

A. Glycosuria is the presence of glucose in urine. (p. 415)

B. Glycosuria is not the presence of glycogen in urine.

C. Glycosuria is not the presence of glucose in blood.

D. Glycosuria is not the presence of glycogen in CSF.

34.

A, C, D. The first step performed in the clean-catch midstream urine collection for women is "After washing her hands, the patient should separate the skin folds around the urinary opening and clean the area."

B. The first step performed in the clean-catch midstream urine collection for women is "After washing her hands, the patient should separate the skin folds around the urinary opening and clean the area." (p. 418)

35.

A. In Figure 15.3, the patient is collecting a sputum specimen (fluid from the lungs containing pus). (pp. 422–423)

B. In Figure 15.3, the patient is not collecting a throat culture specimen.

C. In Figure 15.3, the patient is not collecting a wound specimen.

D. In Figure 15.3, the patient is not collecting a nasopharyngeal culture specimen.

36.

A. The breath analysis test is used to detect peptic ulcers caused by *Helicobacter pylori.*

B. The sweat chloride test is used in the diagnosis of cystic fibrosis. (p. 427)

C. Gastric analysis determines how much acid is produced in an individual's stomach and is not used to detect cystic fibrosis.

D. O & P is a test to detect ova and parasites in fecal specimens.

FIGURE 15.3. Collecting a sterile sputum sample from a patient.

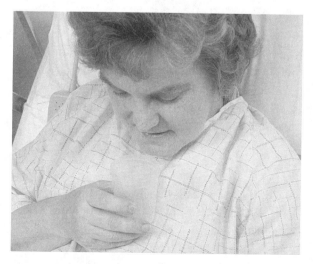

37.

A, C, D. *Helicobacter pylori* is a bacteria that causes peptic ulcers and can be detected through breath analysis.

B. *Helicobacter pylori* is a bacteria that causes peptic ulcers and can be detected through breath analysis. (p. 427)

38.

A. Diabetes mellitus is not a disorder of the exocrine gland that affects the lungs, upper respiratory tract, liver, and pancreas.

B. Cystic fibrosis is a disorder of the exocrine gland that affects the lungs, upper respiratory tract, liver, and pancreas. (p. 427)

C. Pneumonia is not a disorder of the exocrine gland that affects the lungs, upper respiratory tract, liver, and pancreas.

D. Diabetes insipidus is not a disorder of the exocrine gland that affects the lungs, upper respiratory tract, liver, and pancreas.

39.

A. Glycosuria is the presence of glucose in urine.

B. When hemoglobin is detected on the urine dipstick from a patient's urine specimen, this indicates blood destruction with release of free hemoglobin. (p. 415)

C. When hemoglobin is detected on the urine dipstick from a patient's urine specimen, this does not indicate high chloride levels.

D. When hemoglobin is detected on the urine dipstick from a patient's urine specimen, this does not indicate leukocytes in the urine.

40.

A. Glucose level determinations for diabetes mellitus testing should not occur on a random urine specimen.

B. Glucose level determinations for diabetes mellitus testing should occur on a "fasting" urine specimen. (p. 415)

C and D. Glucose level determinations for diabetes mellitus testing should occur on a "fasting" urine specimen.

41.

A. Red blood cells are detected through the chemical analysis of a urine sample.

B. Hemoglobin is detected through the chemical analysis of a urine sample.

C. The "transparency" versus cloudiness is detected through the physical analysis of a urine sample. (pp. 415–416)

D. Ketones are detected through the chemical analysis of a urine sample.

42.

A, B, D. The presence of bilirubin in the urine may be associated with liver disease and obstructive jaundice.

C. The presence of bilirubin in the urine may be associated with liver disease and obstructive jaundice. (p. 415)

43.

A. The "creatinine" clearance test is used to determine the ability of the kidney to remove creatinine from the blood and thus provides information on the kidney's ability to filter analytes from the body. (p. 416)

B. The "creatinine" clearance test, not "creatine," is used to determine the ability of the kidney to remove creatinine from the blood and thus provides information on the kidney's ability to filter analytes from the body. Creatine is an analyte found in the muscles of a person.

C and D. The "creatinine" clearance test is used to determine the ability of the kidney to remove creatinine from the blood and thus provides information on the kidney's ability to filter analytes from the body.

44.

A. Peritoneal fluid is not the fluid collected through a lumbar puncture.

B. Lumbar relates to the spinal vertebrae and thus cerebrospinal fluid is the fluid collected through a lumbar puncture. (p. 419)

C. Lumbar relates to the spinal vertebrae and thus seminal fluid is not the fluid collected through a lumbar puncture.

D. Lumbar relates to the spinal vertebrae and thus pleural fluid is not the fluid collected through a lumbar puncture.

45.

A. The second tube of CSF collected through a spinal tap is not usually used for clinical chemistry testing.

B. The second tube of CSF collected through a spinal tap is not usually used for serological testing.

C. The second tube of CSF collected through a spinal tap is used for clinical microbiology testing. (p. 419)

D. The second tube of CSF collected through a spinal tap is not usually used for microscopic analysis.

46.

A, B, C. When instructing the patient for the collection of a 24-hour urine specimen, if possible, the patient should discontinue medications for 48 to 72 hours preceding the urine collection as a precaution against interference in the laboratory assays.

D. When instructing the patient for the collection of a 24-hour urine specimen, if possible, the patient should discontinue medications for 48 to 72 hours preceding the urine collection as a precaution against interference in the laboratory assays. (p. 420)

47.

A. Fecal specimens are usually not collected to detect *Haemophilus influenzae*.

B. Fecal specimens are sometimes collected in order to detect *Salmonella* species. (p. 421)

C. Fecal specimens are usually not collected to detect *Corynebacterium diphtheriae*.

D. Fecal specimens are usually not collected to detect *Mycobacterium tuberculosis*.

48.

A. The test used to diagnose whooping cough and pneumonia is not a creatinine clearance.

B. The test used to diagnose whooping cough and pneumonia is a nasopharyngeal culture. (p. 423)

C. The test used to diagnose whooping cough and pneumonia is not an O & P.

D. The test used to diagnose whooping cough and pneumonia is not a breath analysis.

49.

A. Seminal fluid is semen collected from a man for various diagnostic procedures.

B. Amniotic fluid is the fluid that bathes the fetus within the amniotic sac.

C. Fluid from the lungs containing pus is sputum. (p. 422)

D. Synovial fluid is fluid surrounding the joints.

50.

A, C, D. In the gastric analysis procedure, histamine is injected into the patient as a stimulant.

B. In the gastric analysis procedure, histamine is injected into the patient as a stimulant. (p. 426)

16 Forensic Toxicology, Workplace Testing, Sports Medicine, and Related Areas

chapter objectives

Upon completion of Chapter 16, the learner is responsible for the following:

➤ Define toxicology and forensic toxicology

➤ Give five examples of specimens that can be used for forensic analysis.

➤ Describe the role of the health care worker or "collector" in federal drug testing programs.

➤ Describe the function of a chain of custody and the Custody and Control Form.

➤ Give examples of situations where drug testing might be valuable.

➤ Describe how to detect adulteration of urine specimens.

DIRECTIONS Each of the questions or incomplete statements below is followed by four suggested answers or completions. Select one answer that is best in each case.

1. "Illicit drugs" include:
   A. alcohol and cigarettes for teens
   B. beer and wine
   C. opiates, cocaine, and amphetamines
   D. all of the above

2. Which drugs are the most commonly used by teenagers?
   A. marijuana
   B. alcohol and tobacco
   C. cocaine and heroin
   D. tranquilizers

3. Among current drug users, what is the most commonly used illicit drug?
   A. alcohol
   B. marijuana
   C. cocaine and heroin
   D. inhalants?

4. Gateway drugs are defined as:
   A. cocaine and opiates
   B. amphetamines
   C. inhalants
   D. alcohol, tobacco, and marijuana

5. The leading cause(s) of death among people aged 15–24 years is/are:
   A. drug overdose
   B. cancer
   C. heart attacks
   D. violence including suicide, homicide, and accidents

6. What does the term "drugged driving" mean?
   A. driving while using chemotherapy
   B. driving while taking steroids
   C. a specific blood alcohol level
   D. driving while under the influence of illicit drugs

7. Which of the following statements defines toxicology?
   A. study and detection of poisons in the body
   B. the study of poisons in urine
   C. legal term meaning illicit drugs
   D. type of specimen that contains toxins

8. Forensic specimens are best described by which of the following statements?
   A. urine or blood specimens that are chemically treated
   B. specimens needed to evaluate liver and kidney function
   C. tissue specimens from a biopsy sample
   D. specimens evaluated for civil or criminal legal cases

9. Which of the following may be forensic specimens in certain circumstances?
   A. bones, nails, and hair
   B. venous and arterial blood
   C. saliva and teeth
   D. all of the above

10. Which of the following statements best defines the chain-of-custody?
    A. parental control process for teenagers who abuse drugs
    B. process for maintaining control of specimens from collection to delivery
    C. specimen transportation vehicle for clinical laboratories
    D. metal chain that is used to lock specimens in a tamper-proof safe

11. A chain-of-custody form must contain the identification of a subject, the time and date of the sample collection, and:
    A. a tamper-evident seal
    B. the signature of the subject or patient
    C. the name of the individual who obtained the specimen
    D. all of the above

12. After a specimen reaches its destination, the chain-of-custody process requires that:
    A. an armed guard be on the premises during testing phases and sign-in as a witness
    B. the specimen is never opened to violate the tamper-evident seal
    C. the specimen handler must sign and complete the chain-of-custody form
    D. the donor of the specimen be present

13. The listed acronyms indicate a federal agency and a document that is important to drug testing for federal employees. Identify the correct names for the following: DOT and CCF.
    A. Department of Transportation and the Custody and Control Form
    B. Department of Toxicology and the Center for Criminal Forensics
    C. Department of Transportation and the Center for Custody Forms

D. Division of Testing and the Custody and Control Form

14. Professional sports associations such as the National Basketball Association (NBA) and the National Football League (NFL) are among the organizations that have adopted drug-screening programs for their employees. Which of the following statements is *not* accurate in relation to drug-testing employees in these organizations?
    A. Employees have no rights to privacy.
    B. Procedures for collection and testing are well defined.
    C. Employees being tested must initial the specimen label or seal it.
    D. Screening is often done without prior notice to the employee.

15. What is "blood doping"?
    A. serum levels of marijuana
    B. level of marijuana that produces physical or judgmental impairment
    C. use of blood or blood substitutes to improve endurance
    D. use of steroids

16. Select the organization that performs over 10,000 drug tests annually on its members.
    A. JCAHO
    B. NCAA
    C. ASCP
    D. NCCLS

17. When is workplace drug testing appropriate?
    A. to comply with federal reglations
    B. to enforce a policy of "no drug use"
    C. to comply with contract or insurance requirements
    D. all of the above

18. What is indicated when an employee undergoes drug testing "for cause"?

    A. It means that trace amounts of a drug have been identified.

    B. It is part of every preemployment physical in the country.

    C. It means that the employee showed signs of being impaired or undergoing unsafe work practices.

    D. It means that the employee did not cause the error in question.

19. DNA testing is often used for forensic purposes to:

    A. track criminals released on probation

    B. determine the cause of death

    C. confirm identity

    D. detect drug levels

20. According to guidelines for federal workplace testing programs, what happens if the specimen collector cannot ensure the specimen integrity?

    A. The process should be completed and documented.

    B. He or she will have to track down the donor to collect another specimen.

    C. He or she will be banned from collecting other specimens.

    D. The specimen and test results cannot be considered a valid piece of evidence.

21. Which are steps that can be taken for security measures at sites where specimens for drug screening are collected?

    A. Bluing agents must be added to the toilet bowl accessed by the donor.

    B. Taking the temperature of the urine specimen.

    C. Access to water during the urine collection procedure should be restricted.

    D. All of the above.

22. After a urine sample has been collected for drug testing and the donor gives it to the health care worker, what is the *first* thing the health care worker should do?

    A. Thank the donor for his or her time and escort the donor out.

    B. Read the specimen temperature within 4 minutes.

    C. Check for evidence of drug abuse.

    D. Take fingerprints of the donor.

23. In drug testing, why would a urine specimen temperature need to be taken after collection?

    A. To check for infectious bacteria.

    B. Because some illicit drugs raise the temperature of urine.

    C. To check for evidence of tampering.

    D. To check for fever in the donor.

24. Circumstances under which a specimen for drug testing might be rejected include which of the following?

    A. The donor's signature is not present.

    B. The chain-of-custody was not signed.

    C. The seal is missing or shows evidence of tampering.

    D. All of the above.

25. Which of the following steps can ruin a laboratory result in collecting blood for alcohol levels?

    A. cleansing the site with alcohol

    B. talking with the specimen donor

    C. vein selection on the appropriate arm

    D. labeling the specimen so that it cannot be viewed

26. How is forensic laboratory analysis different from other types of laboratory testing?
    A. Specimens may be exposed to rain, mud, or mixed with other human tissues.
    B. Specimens always involve illicit drug use.
    C. Specimens must be identified.
    D. Specimens become the property of the federal government.

27. Alcohol intoxication is defined by:
    A. blood alcohol concentration in grams per deciliter
    B. whether or not the individual can walk and talk at the same time
    C. urine alcohol levels
    D. how clearly the individual can communicate

28. The legal limit of alcohol adopted by most states is:
    A. 0.05
    B. 0.08
    C. 1.00
    D. 2.0

29. A common test method used primarily by law enforcement officials to detect alcohol intoxication is:
    A. a metal detector
    B. a hair testing device
    C. an evidential breath testing device
    D. a specific gravity device

30. What specimen is most commonly used for detection of neonatal drug exposure?
    A. hair
    B. sputum
    C. blood
    D. urine

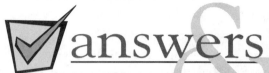

answers & rationales

1.

A. Alcohol and cigarette use by teens is not considered illicit, even though such use is harmful and illegal in many cases.

B. Beer and wine are not defined as illicit drugs.

C. Illicit drugs include opiates, cocaine, amphetamines, and others. (p. 432)

D. "All of the above" is incorrect.

2.

A.–D. The most commonly used drugs by teenagers are alcohol and tobacco. (p. 432)

3.

A. Alcohol is not categorized as an illicit drug.

B. Marijuana is the most commonly used illicit drug (used by 76% of current illicit drug users. (p. 432)

C. Cocaine and heroin are not as widely used as marijuana.

D. Inhalants are not as widely used as marijuana.

4.

A. Cocaine and opiates are illicit drugs and are not usually considered gateway drugs.

B. Amphetamines are illicit drugs and are not usually considered gateway drugs.

C. Inhalants are not usually considered gateway drugs.

D. Gateway drugs are alcohol, tobacco, and marijuana. Adolescents with substance abuse problems tend to begin with alcohol and cigarettes, progress to marijuana, and then move on to using other drugs or combinations of drugs. (p. 432)

5.

A. The leading causes of death among people ages 15–24 years are not drug overdoses.

B. The leading causes of death among people ages 15–24 years are not cancer-related.

C. The leading causes of death among people ages 15–24 years are not heart attacks.

D. The leading causes of death among people ages 15–24 years are acts of violence, including accidents, suicides, and homicides. (p. 432)

6.

A. Drugged driving does not mean "while using chemotherapy."

B. Drugged driving does not mean " while taking steroids."

C. Drugged driving does not refer to a specific blood alcohol level.

D. Drugged driving means driving while under the influence of illicit drugs. (p. 432)

7.

A. Toxicology is defined as the scientific study of poisons, how they are detected, how they react in the body, and the treatment of the conditions they produce. (p. 433)

B. Toxicology may include the study of poisons in urine; however, the definition is much broader.

C. Toxicology is not a legal term meaning illicit drugs.

D. Toxicology is not a type of specimen that contains toxins.

8.

A. There are many other specimens that can be forensic specimens besides urine and blood, and they are not necessarily "chemically treated."

B. Forensic specimens are not specimens needed to evaluate liver and kidney function in a normal patient.

C. Forensic specimens are not necessarily tissue specimens from a biopsy sample, although they may be in certain circumstances.

D. Forensic specimens are those involved in and evaluated for civil or criminal legal cases. (p. 433)

9.

A.–D. (The correct answer is D.) The following may be forensic specimens in certain circumstances: saliva, teeth, bones, nails, hair, venous, capillary, and arterial blood, clothing, dried blood stains, sperm, sweat, and urine. (p. 433)

10.

A. Chain-of-custody does not refer to a parental control process for teenagers who abuse drugs.

B. The chain-of-custody is a process for maintaining control of specimens from the time of sample collection to delivery or final disposition of the specimen. (p. 434)

C. Chain-of-custody does not refer to a specimen transportation vehicle for clinical laboratories.

D. Chain-of-custody does not refer to a metal chain for locking specimens.

11.

A.–D. (The correct answer is D.) A chain-of-custody form must contain the identification of a subject, the time and date of the sample collection, the name of the health care worker who obtained and processed the specimen, the signature of the subject or patient, and a tamper-evident seal. (pp. 437–438)

12.

A. An armed guard is not necessary on the premises during testing phases.

B. The specimen must be opened for testing purposes, so the tamper-evident seal will be broken. This is part of the normal process, however, documentation for the chain-of-custody must be maintained.

C. After a specimen reaches its destination, the chain-of-custody process requires that the individual who handles the specimen or an aliquot of the specimen must sign and complete the chain-of-custody form. (pp. 437–438)

D. The donor of the specimen will not likely be present at the time the specimen reaches its destination.

13.

A. The acronyms DOT and CCF stand for Department of Transportation, a federal agency, and the Custody and Control Form, a chain-of-custody document that is important to drug testing for federal employees. Standards have been published by the DOT relating to the testing of specimens, quality assurance and quality control, chain-of-custody, personnel, and how results are reported for federal drug testing programs. (p. 435)

B. The acronyms DOT and CCF do not represent Department of Toxicology and the Center for Criminal Forensics.

C. The acronym DOT stands for the Department of Transportation, but CCF does not represent the Center for Custody Forms.

D. The acronym CCF stands for the Custody and Control Form, but DOT does not stand for Division of Testing.

14.

A. All individuals have a right to privacy. Privacy is important in the specimen collection process, however, if there is a suspicion of tampering with the specimen, privacy may be somewhat compromised. (p. 439)

B.–D. Drug testing employees in organizations such as the NBA and the NFL usually involves screening without prior notice to the employee, procedures for collection and testing are well defined, and the employee being tested must initial the specimen label or seal.

15.

A.–B. The term "blood doping" does not relate to marijuana use.

C. "Blood doping" refers to the practice of injecting red cells, whole blood, or blood substitutes to increase endurance and oxygen-carrying capacity of the blood. It has been done by athletes, particularly in endurance sports such as cycling. It is also associated with cardiovascular problems. (p. 439)

D. The term "blood doping" does not relate to steroid use.

16.

A. JCAHO does not perform over 10,000 drug tests annually on its members.

B. The National Collegiate Athletic Association (NCAA) performs over 10,000 drug tests annually on its members. (p. 439)

C. ASCP does not perform over 10,000 drug tests annually on its members.

D. NCCLS does not perform over 10,000 drug tests annually on its members.

17.

A.–D. (The correct answer is D.) Workplace drug testing is appropriate to comply with federal regulations, with customer or contract requirements, insurance carrier requirements, to reinforce the policy of "no drug use" to identify users and refer them for assistance, to minimize the chances of hiring employees who are drug users, and to improve safety. (p. 435)

18.

A. It does not indicate that trace amounts of a drug have been identified.

B. It is not a part of every preemployment physical in the country.

C. It means that the employer is requesting the drug test because the employee showed signs of being impaired or undergoing unsafe work practices. (p. 435)

D. It does not relate to causes of an unspecified error.

19.

A. DNA testing is not often used for tracking criminals on probation.

B. DNA testing is not used to determine the cause of death in forensic cases.

C. DNA testing is used to confirm identity in forensic cases because it is very accurate. (p. 434)

D. DNA testing is not used to detect drug levels.

20.

A. If a specimen collector cannot ensure the donor specimen's integrity, the process should be discontinued and appropriate documentation filed.

B. Usually the specimen collector is not responsible for "tracking down the donor."

C. Depending on the circumstances, the specimen collector may be accountable for the consequences of poor specimen integrity. However, it is unlikely that he or she would be "banned."

D. If a specimen collector cannot ensure the donor specimen's integrity, the specimen and test results cannot be considered a valid piece of evidence. (p. 437)

21.

A.–D. (The correct answer is D.) Security measures at sites where specimens for drug screening are collected involve use of bluing agents in the toilet bowl accessed by the donor (to determine whether or not the donor has diluted the urine specimen with toilet water), restricted access to water during the urine collection procedure, taking the temperature of the urine specimen, and secure handling and storage so that the donor need not carry in large bags or articles that can be used to hide a specimen (to substitute for the real one); only collection sup- plies should be taken into the collection stall. (p. 437)

22.

A. The donor should not be allowed to leave until all checks have been made, the specimen has been sealed, initials have been acquired, and the Custody and Control Form has been completed.

B. The specimen temperature should be read within 4 minutes for evidence of tampering. (p. 437)

C. The health care worker is not responsible for checking for evidence of drug abuse.

D. The health care worker is not responsible for taking fingerprints.

23.

A. Urine temperature does not assess the presence or absence of infectious bacteria.

B. Illicit drug use alone does not raise the temperature of urine.

C. In drug testing, a urine specimen temperature is taken after collection to check for evidence of tampering. Donors who worry about detection of drugs in their urine may want to dilute the sample with water or other fluids. Normally, fresh urine has a normal body temperature. If cold water (from the toilet or other source) is added to the urine, it will not be at the correct temperature, and tampering is suspected. If this is the case, the health care worker may request another specimen under direct observation according to federal guidelines. (p. 437)

D. Urine temperature does not assess fever in the donor.

24.

A.–D. (The correct answer is D.) Circumstances under which a specimen for drug testing might be rejected include that the donor's signature is not present and there is no indication that the donor refused, the seal is missing or shows evidence of tampering, the chain-of-custody was not signed by the collector, there is insufficient quantity, there has obviously been tampering with the specimen, there is an identification problem, or there is mismatched documentation. (pp. 436–438)

25.

A. Cleansing the site with alcohol can ruin a laboratory result when collecting blood for alcohol levels if the health care worker is not careful. A nonalcoholic disinfectant should be used to cleanse the site to avoid contamination of the specimen with the alcoholic disinfectant. (p. 441)

B. This answer is not appropriate.

C. Vein selection on the appropriate arm will not interfere with the test.

D. Labeling the specimen so that it cannot be viewed should not normally interfere with the test.

26.

A. Forensic laboratory analysis differs from other types of clinical laboratory testing because the specimens may have been exposed to rain, mud, or may be mixed with other individuals' specimens. (p. 434)

B. Forensic analysis does not "always involve illicit drug use."

C. Specimens must be correctly identified whether they are for forensic or clinical laboratory testing.

D. Forensic specimens do not necessarily become the "property of the federal government."

27.

A. Alcohol intoxication is defined by blood alcohol concentration in grams per deciliter. (p. 440)

B. Alcohol intoxication is not defined by whether or not the individual can walk and talk simultaneously.

C. Alcohol intoxication is not defined by urine alcohol levels.

D. Alcohol intoxication is not defined by how clearly an individual can communicate.

28.

A, C, D. The following levels are *not* the "legal limits" of alcohol intoxication: 0.05, 1.00, 2.0. Even though these levels and not part of the "legal" definition, impaired functioning may occur, especially in the *higher* levels.

B. The legal limit now adopted by most states is 0.08 (0.08 grams of alcohol per 100 ml of blood). (p. 440)

29.

A. A metal detector does not detect alcohol intoxication.

B. A hair testing device does not detect alcohol intoxication.

C. A common test method used primarily by law enforcement officials to detect alcohol intoxication is an evidential breath testing (EBT) analyzer. (p. 440)

D. A specific gravity device does not detect alcohol intoxication.

30.

A. Hair is not used for detection of neonatal drug exposure.

B. Sputum is not used for detection of neonatal drug exposure.

C. Blood is not as commonly used for detection of neonatal drug exposure.

D. Urine is commonly used for detection of neonatal drug exposure. (p. 441)

Index